Hormone Re Meal Plan

21 Day Hormone Reset Plan

Jessica Billings

Introduction

Have you been experiencing chronic anxiety, almost-constant cravings, sluggishness, a lagging libido, stress, weight gain, stubborn belly fat lately? You are most probably suffering from hormone imbalance. You may have sought conventional help from doctors who prescribe you creams, pills and shots. These are highly ineffective as they only treat the symptoms that manifest on the surface but the root problem underneath persists.

What you need, my friend, is an individualized approach to reset the efficacy of your seven metabolic hormones namely estrogen, insulin, leptin, growth hormone, testosterone, thyroid and cortisol. Developing resistance to these hormones slows down your metabolism and leads to weight gain and sluggishness. The Hormone Reset Diet is a plan that's specially designed for women from all walks of life to lose weight and feel more energetic.

You will have to eliminate some types of foods (that wreck havoc and develop resistance to your major metabolic hormones) and substitute them for more hormone friendly foods. By making simple dietary changes, you will be able to reverse hormone resistance, rebalance hormone receptors and enhance metabolism to kick start weight loss in only 3 weeks.

Are you ready to start get past your weight loss plateau? If you are, let this book mark the end of your weight loss struggles for good!

In this book, you will learn:

- Why your weight problems may have another cause
- What this other cause may be
- The place of hormones in determining your weight
- How a hormone reset may be your express ticket to effortless weight loss
- How to reset different hormones to restore your health and lose weight effortlessly
- How to reset your hormones
- Delicious hormone reset diet recipes you can prepare for the next 3 weeks to realize weight loss and other health benefits
- And much more!

By reading this book and taking action, your weight loss struggles will be a thing of the past.

Let's begin!

Table of Contents

Introduction _____ 2

What Are Hormones? _____ 8

The 9 Metabolic Hormones & How Their Imbalance Results To Weight Gain _____ 9

How To Reset Leptin _____ 22

Self-Assessment _____ 22

How To Reset The Leptin Hormone _____ 24

How To Reset Cortisol _____ 27

Self-Assessment _____ 27

How To Reset Cortisol _____ 28

How To Reset Insulin _____ 32

Self-Assessment _____ 32

How To Reset Insulin _____ 33

How To Reset Estrogen Dominance — 41

Self-Assessment — 41

How To Reset Estrogen — 42

How To Reset Thyroid — 49

Self-Assessment — 49

How To Reset The Thyroid — 50

How To Reset Testosterone — 57

Self-Assessment — 57

How To Reset Testosterone — 58

How To Reset Your Growth Hormone — 63

Self-Assessment — 63

How To Reset Your Growth Hormone — 64

Hormone Reset Recipes — 70

Shakes And Smoothies — 70

Kale And Sunflower Smoothie — 75

Breakfast Recipes _____ *78*

Lunch Recipes _____ *92*

Dinner Recipes _____ *114*

21 Day Hormone Reset Plan _____ **136**

Conclusion _____ **142**

Hormone Imbalance And Weight Gain

Before we get a point of learning how to reset your hormones to bring about weight loss and other benefits, let's start by understanding the basics first, starting with:

What Are Hormones?

Hormones are simply molecules or 'special chemical messengers' (that are secreted by special glands e.g. the adrenal glands) within the body's endocrine system. The function of hormones is to regulate various biological functions such as electrolyte and water balance, storage and energy use, development, reproduction and growth. Most hormones are carried by the circulatory system to all parts of the body where they affect the tissues and cells as necessary.

However, specific hormones only influence the target cells that have receptors for every specific hormone. For that reason, when a hormone binds to a cell **receptor**, some change takes place within the cell to bring about a particular cellular function. This is what **hormone signaling** is all about.

Sometimes though, hormonal imbalance is as a result of poor lifestyle choices and this ultimately leads to unhealthy weight gain. Listed below are some of the major metabolic hormones and how their imbalance results in weight gain:

The 9 Metabolic Hormones & How Their Imbalance Results To Weight Gain

Leptin

Leptin is commonly referred to as the satiety hormone. It is produced by the stored fat cells of the white adipose tissues.

This means that the amount of leptin released into your bloodstream is directly in proportion to the entire amount of fat in your body. Thus, the more fat in your body, the greater the amount of leptin you produce.

Leptin is a very essential hormone when it comes to understanding your feelings of satiety and hunger. When its level is low, you begin to feel hungry or begin to crave for food. When produced in high quantities however, it signals the brain to tell you that you have had enough food and should stop eating.

Low leptin levels stimulate the hypothalamus to produce some chemicals namely NPY (neuropeptide Y) and anandamide, which are both strong feeding stimulants and they drive up your hunger levels. On the contrary, high leptin levels also stimulate the hypothalamus to produce another chemical known as alpha-MSH (alpha-Melanocyte stimulating hormone) which is an appetite suppressant and it makes you feel satiated such that you no longer feel like eating.

People who are obese or overweight have more body fat in their fat cells than necessary. Since fat cells are the ones that secrete leptin in proportion to the amount of body fat, such persons tend to have very high amounts of leptin in the blood.

Considering the way in which leptin works, and given the brain knows that the body has more than enough energy reserves, such people shouldn't actually eat. However, the excessive levels of leptin being produced mess up with the signaling and detection mechanism such that the brain no longer senses the presence of leptin. This phenomenon is what we refer to as **leptin resistance.**

Leptin resistance happens when your body is continuously overexposed to high levels of leptin and it eventually affects your brain's sensitivity to leptin. When your body becomes resistant to leptin, it may require a much higher quantity of leptin before the brain signals the body that you feel full. So obese persons have abnormally high leptin levels but they are unresponsive to it. This explains their almost insatiable appetite and constant cravings.

Ghrelin

Also commonly known as the hunger hormone, ghrelin is a peptide hormone that is secreted by the ghrelinergic cells that are found in the gastrointestinal tract (stomach) and its function is to stimulate appetite.

Ghrelin is produced when your stomach is empty. Once it is produced, ghrelin, just like leptin, crosses the blood-brain barrier and finds its way to your hypothalamus to alert you that you are hungry. Ghrelin also plays a role in deposition of fat around the body. The pancreas, small intestines and brain also produce ghrelin but in smaller quantities.

Thus, ghrelin levels are lowest when you have eaten and are high just before you eat. However, in obese and/or overweight people, ghrelin levels are abnormally lower than in people with normal weight. When an overweight person is eating, ghrelin only drops off slightly. As a result, the hypothalamus fails to receive as strong a message as it should to stop you from eating and you end up overfeeding.

What is more, ghrelin is secreted directly in response to a stressful situation. This explains why so many people have the tendency to over-eat when they're stressed out. Ghrelin brings about weight gain by perpetuating the stress cycle. Ghrelin is produced in order to try and maintain your stress levels and this causes the side effects of having strong urges to overeat.

Cortisol

Cortisol, which is also popularly known as the stress hormone is a form of a steroid hormone and is secreted by the adrenal glands, which are endocrine glands found just above the kidney.

Cortisol is a fight or flight hormone that is secreted when you are stressed out, anxious, angry, depressed, nervous or physically injured. It is produced so as to replenish the energy you expend after fleeing from or fighting off a perceived threat. Poor lifestyle choices and inadequate sleep also makes your body be in a constant state of stress.

But too often, the modern human being usually responds to stress by stewing and sitting in sadness, anger or frustration without using up any energy that you would have if you were physically fleeing or fighting a wild beast hunting you down (like our ancestors so often did).

And so while you are seated there wallowing in stressful thoughts, your neuro-endocrine system believes that you are physically fleeing or fighting. Nonetheless, cortisol is still released into your system whether or not your stressor requires you to respond physically or emotionally.

For some people, cortisol runs through their bodies almost constantly since their typical day has no break from stress. This makes their bodies' 'hyper-insulinemic' and it increases the deposition of fat on the body. This constantly elevated cortisol also leaves you vulnerable to developing conditions such high blood pressure, diabetes and in general lowers your immunity.

Melatonin

To maintain your body's internal clock (when you sleep and wake up); melatonin is secreted by a pea-shaped gland located in your brain known as the pineal gland.

Melatonin affects your body's daily cycles such as body temperature, sleep and metabolism through feedback communication between the hormone producing glands and the brain. Secretion of melatonin takes place mostly during the night because light has been found to somehow hinder the production of this hormone. This means that melatonin levels are lowest during daytime.

Age is also a factor in melatonin synthesis. According to the journal of clinical pharmacology, the production of melatonin is very low between the ages of 6 and 20 but then stabilizes between 20s and 40s after then begins to drop again once you've gone past 40.

Researchers have found that there is a link between low levels of melatonin and a tendency to put on weight. In a study titled 'endocrinology' published in December 2013, it was shown that surgically removing the pineal gland caused weight gain in rats. The same study also shows how obese rats lost weight after getting melatonin supplementation without having to change their food consumption.

Getting some quality rest at night is not easy when insufficient melatonin is being produced. If you keep disrupting your circadian rhythm either because it is not dark enough around or for some reason you cannot get enough sleep, you increase the production of leptin, ghrelin and cortisol. Once these hormones are released into the bloodstream in high doses, you end up gaining weight and you also make losing the weight way more difficult.

Thyroid Hormones

Thyroid hormones are produced by the thyroid gland, which is butterfly shaped and is located at the back of your neck. The 3 most active thyroid hormones produced are triiodothyronine (T3), thyroxine (T4), and calcitonin. These three work together to regulate your body's metabolic functioning, bone maintenance, mood regulation, brain development, muscle control as well as heart and digestive functions.

Underproduction of these thyroid hormones (hypothyroidism) is strongly associated with gaining weight. In fact, sudden weight gain is one of the most common signs that the thyroid is not producing enough hormones. Studies show that hypothyroidism affects one woman in five and in over half of these cases, this condition is not diagnosed.

Nutrient deficiencies, stress and physical inactivity are some of the reasons for an underperforming thyroid. Others include environmental toxins such as pesticides and heavy metals e.g. mercury. Gluten intolerance also plays a major role in hypothyroidism. It is also said that hypothyroidism also leads to accumulation of water in the body making a patient appear plump. For your thyroid to run optimally you need to include sufficient omega 3 fatty acids, iodine, zinc and selenium to your diet.

Estrogen

Estrogen is one of the two main sex hormones found in women and is produced in the ovarian cells. Any estrogen imbalance, whether low or high, will cause weight gain. This is why it needs to be maintained at an optimum.

High levels of estrogen can be caused when you consume a diet that is rich in estrogen e.g. red meat. Nowadays, beef cattle are fed with synthetic estrogen compounds such as estrogen pellets to improve their feeding efficiency and enable them to pack on more weight so that the farmer may fetch handsome profits once they are sold.

Other culprits include consuming too much alcohol, refined carbs and sugar. There are also xenoestrogens. These are synthetic or natural chemicals that mimic the structural parts of estrogen compounds and therefore exert estrogenic effects in your body. Most xenoestrogens are found in chemicals, pesticides, plastics and water systems.

Increased estrogen stresses the cells that produce insulin in your body. You therefore end up becoming insulin resistant and blood sugar levels go high and then you end up gaining weight. Other than gaining weight, other symptoms of estrogen imbalance are heavy menstrual bleeding, fibroids, fluid retention and breast tenderness.

Women who are at their pre-menopausal stage are also at risk. At this stage, the ovarian cells secrete less estrogen and since there isn't enough supply of estrogen anymore, the body resorts to other sources such as fat cells. The body begins to convert all the available sources of energy to fat so as to replenish glucose levels. Eventually, you end up packing on weight especially in the lower abdomen area. Women between the ages of 35 and 50 are at the highest risk since their ovaries secrete less progesterone and thus allowing estrogen to take over.

Testosterone

This steroidal hormone is produced by humans beings and animals alike. It is predominantly a male sex hormone even though females produce it too but in little amounts.

Testosterone is the hormone responsible for increased muscle mass, bone density, libido, facial hair and even deep voice. In other words, testosterone is imperative for a healthy body and plays a vital role in metabolism.

Studies show that people with low testosterone have a higher percentage of body fat as compared to people with higher quantities of testosterone. This means that a dip in testosterone levels causes an increase in body weight especially in the midsection (and the opposite is true). Researchers are not quite sure why testosterone levels are lower in overweight people but research points to the following:

Belly fat has the highest level of enzyme aromatase whose function is to convert testosterone into estrogen. This could explain why overweight people have high estrogen levels than normal. In addition, this estrogen and aromatase activity decreases the secretion of GRH (Gonadotropin releasing hormone). Insufficient GRH causes the drop in the production of luteinizing hormone, which in turn leads to the reduction in the production of testosterone.

Age and stress are some of the reasons behind low testosterone production. Inadequate exercise, irregular sleep patterns and poor diet are other causes. Being overweight hinders your body's ability to produce enough testosterone and further lowers the already low testosterone level in the body and this can spiral into a vicious cycle.

Insulin

Insulin is released by your pancreas (an organ in your abdomen) and its purpose is to help carry glucose into the cells so that it can be used as energy or to be converted and stored as fat. Think of the hormone insulin as a key that you use to unlock the cell doors so that glucose may enter. In short, insulin helps maintain a healthy level of glucose in the blood.

Blood sugar levels go up as you eat. Insulin lowers it from the bloodstream by directing it into 3 different organs of your body to avoid the glucose levels going beyond the normal range. Most of the glucose is used up by the muscles as fuel, a little amount of it is directed to the liver, and the rest is converted and stored as fat.

Some poor lifestyle choices such as binging on alcohol, artificially sweetened drinks and poor diet, processed foods and snacking leads to insulin resistance. This is a phenomenon where the cell receptors are no longer sensitive to or no longer respond to insulin, even though the hormone is there in plenty. This means that cells no longer acknowledge the presence of the glucose-bound insulin thus, glucose remains in the bloodstream. This spike in blood sugar levels leads to Type 2 diabetes and a sudden weight gain. Too much fat within the pancreas and the liver disrupts normal insulin production and action. Both of these defects however are reversible by losing a considerable amount of weight.

Human Growth Hormone

The Human Growth Hormone (HGH), also known simply as the Growth Hormone (GH), is produced by the pituitary gland. Its function is to boost metabolism, cell production and repair, body composition and muscle growth.

HGH is recorded at its highest point in persons at their mid 20s but begins to gradually decline in the early 40s. Optimum HGH helps you recover from disease and injury and boosts your exercise performance and strength. Sufficient HGH in your body is especially important during weight loss, as it increases the breakdown of triglycerides (stored fat) to be used as body fuel.

However, low levels of HGH have been linked to weight gain. Other than that, low HGH also increases the risk of developing disease (low immunity) and in general, it negatively affects the quality of life. Unsurprisingly, studies have shown that poor diet and lifestyle choices are the major factors in HGH deficiency.

Studies show that the production of HGH is directly related to the amount of your body fat. The more visceral fat or the higher the body fat content you have in general means that you are likely to have an impaired production of HGH, and thus an increased risk of developing disease. In one study for instance, it was discovered that persons who had about three times the amount of belly fat as the control group had less than half the required amount of HGH. In another study, overweight persons were found to have lower amounts of HGH and IGF-1 which is also a growth related hormone. However, after they went through a process of losing a significant amount of their weight, their HGH and IGF-1 levels became normal once more.

Next, we will discuss how to reset each of the 7 hormones to kick-start your weight loss journey.

How To Reset Leptin

Self-Assessment

Most of these signs may not necessarily mean that you are resistant to leptin but it should be a cause for concern if you happen to experience more than 4 of these symptoms. If that is the case, there are chances that you are might be leptin resistant and you should visit a doctor for serum blood testing.

The doctor may review your history of illness and assess your symptoms before taking a blood sample for further tests to determine your leptin levels. Depending on how the results pan out, the doctor can make a diagnosis or recommend further tests because leptin levels may vary from one day to another. Therefore, the doctor can advise you to visit again to check leptin levels for diagnosis. The optimum serum leptin level should be below 10 – 12. If it is greater than that and you are no less than 9 kgs (20 pounds) overweight, then you may be leptin resistant.

A person with leptin resistance may have no less than 4 of the following signs:

Hormone Reset Diet Meal Plan

- Continuous weight gain and a voracious appetite

- Difficulty in losing weight even after exercising regularly and dieting

- Uncontrolled food cravings for sweet and salty junk foods even after having a huge meal

- A diagnosis of insulin resistance or metabolic syndrome

- Fatigue or having low energy or feeling sluggish

- Deteriorating complications of hydrothyroidism (a condition in which your thyroid glands don't produce enough thyroid hormones) such as joint pains, infertility, obesity etc.

- Cold body temperatures, which are less than 36°C or 98°F.

- Slow resting heart rate (below 60) which is a result of poor aerobic conditioning and being overweight or obese

- Reduced sex drive and infertility

To reverse leptin resistance you need to do the following:

How To Reset The Leptin Hormone

Eliminate Fructose Completely

Fructose is a simple natural sugar found in honey, fruits and vegetables as well as food and drink sweeteners such as high fructose corn syrup. Fructose is also the major component in brown sugar, table sugar, agave, maple syrup and molasses. Carbonated cola for instance contains about 30 grams of fructose.

Around 60% of the world adult population has the limited ability to absorb fructose and get it converted into and stored as fat.

Fructose causes the hypothalamus to be resistant to leptin. The normal functioning receptors in the hypothalamus seem to be ineffective and muted in the presence of leptin when fructose level in the blood is high. Moreover, high fructose consumption results in the body producing a lot of triglycerides.

Triglycerides are known to block the passageway of leptin to the brain. Studies show that triglycerides encourage leptin resistance by impairing the transport of leptin across the blood brain barrier. This means that the leptin reaching the receptors in the brain is insufficient to produce the effect desired.

Don't Snack After Dinner

Let dinner be the last meal of the day; period. Make sure that you have a minimum of 3 hours after eating dinner before you go to bed. Never go to bed on a full stomach. Also, make sure that you maintain 11-12 hours between dinner and breakfast. Leptin levels rise and fall on a regular rhythm that follows a 24 hour pattern. It has been observed that levels of leptin peak at the evening hours.

This happens so that the body may undergo nighttime self repair and recovery. It is leptin that coordinates the timing and production of hormone melatonin, which allows for entrainment (synchronization) of the circadian rhythm, metabolism and body rejuvenation while sleeping. But all this will happen if you do not eat or snack at all after dinner.

Cold Therapy

Yes, that's correct and if you are wondering know, exposing yourself to cold temperatures has many health benefits. First of all, it can aid in speedy recovery from injury especially (muscle injuries), reduce pain threshold, improve your bone health, improve the quality of your sleep, enhance your immune system, and even increase your lifespan etc. even more surprising is that it can help you shed off a few pounds.

Studies show that the leptin receptors are more efficient when you expose yourself to cold temperatures. Therefore, cold therapy can reverse insulin resistance by increasing leptin sensitivity.

Cold therapy is actually very simple as you can even do it in the comfort of your home by turning down your house's thermostat. You can also bath in a bathtub filled with cold water or you can swim in cold water. Also, there are crycotherapy iceboxes that are mostly used in the field of sports medicine.

How To Reset Cortisol

Self-Assessment

You need to reset your cortisol if you meet at least 4 of the criteria below:

- Strangely enough, perhaps that the more coffee/caffeinated drink you take, the more sluggish and tired you become once the 'caffeine buzz' wears off.
- Dependency, tolerance or addiction to coffee
- Premenstrual syndrome (PMS)
- Physical or emotional exhaustion or burnout due to chronic stress
- Anxiety or irritability struggles
- A tendency to overeat when stressed
- Problem falling asleep at night
- Breast tenderness or any fibrocystic breast changes
- Regular gastroesophagial reflux disease, stomach ulcers or indigestion

- Osteopenia or osteoporosis (thinning bones)

How To Reset Cortisol

To stabilize cortisol levels in your blood, you need to do the following:

Eliminate Coffee Or Caffeine Related Products Completely -

Did you know that 75% to 80% of the world's population drinks coffee or other caffeinated beverages on a regular basis? In addition, about 80% of adult Americans consume coffee regularly every day. For most people, having a sizzling cup of coffee first thing after waking up is a comforting ritual that marks the start of a new day.

Caffeine (whose scientific name is 1,3,7-trimethylxanthine) acts as a stimulant to the central nervous system and produces some 'happy' effects in the brain. People drink coffee as a way to improve their wakefulness and alertness, mental focus and improve their energy every morning to face the challenges that the new day brings with it.

But while caffeine offers these amazing benefits, it could also spike the levels of the stress hormone cortisol. There is also a strong relationship between elevated levels of cortisol and obesity and especially around the midsection. Other than promoting excess storage of fat, chronically high levels of cortisol can cause catabolic, muscle breakdown in the body. According to a study published in the International Journal of Sports Nutrition and Exercise Metabolism, consuming high levels of caffeine can result in a lower testosterone to cortisol ratio. This effect could potentially offset any anabolic building of muscle.

A typical cup of coffee contains about 100 mg of caffeine per cup. Continued high doses of caffeine between 750 mg to 1,200 mg per day could lead you to develop tolerance to the drug and chronic high levels of cortisol. Tolerance means that it gets to a point when you have increase the amount of coffee you take per day to maintain the same level of alertness and focus throughout a period of time. Indeed, if your system is so dependent and used to a regular dose of coffee, you may suffer some nasty symptoms such as headaches, poor concentration, fatigue and anxiety when you abruptly stop taking the drug.

Eliminate all coffee and caffeinated products such as regular tea, black tea, hot chocolate, sodas, energy drinks, green tea and for good. Did you also know that kola nuts and cocoa beans are some of the most common sources of caffeine?

Replace these with much healthier alternatives such as herbal teas, hot water with cardamom, hot water with cayenne and lemon and mushroom teas, etc.

Exercise Regularly

Studies conducted by researchers from the Harvard Medical School revealed that 30 minutes or an hour of exercise a few times each week is the best way to manage stress because it balances cortisol levels. Exercise normalizes your metabolic functions and helps you sleep better.

But don't forget that too much of everything is dangerous. Many people with leptin resistance make the mistake of overtraining so that they can lose more weight in a short span of time. What they don't know is that in doing so, they make it even the more difficult for them to shed a few pounds and here's why. Pushing your training regimen beyond the set limit raises your cortisol levels due to the stress that you exert on your body. High cortisol levels can alter your insulin levels and consequently, making weight loss difficult to achieve.

Also, it is important to time your workouts well. It is best to work out in the morning or in the mid afternoon if you are looking for a great energy boost. Avoid working out in the evening or during the night. Such late workouts may be doing more harm than good to your cortisol levels if they prompt anxiety or insomnia when you should be asleep.

How To Reset Insulin

Self-Assessment

You need to reset your insulin if you meet at least 4 of the criteria below:

- Blood sugar level is higher than it should i.e. if it is higher than 85 milligrams per deciliter.

- You try to quit eating candies and other sweet stuff without any degree of success. In simple terms, you can't stop eating foods packed in carbs such as ice cream, chocolate or even French fries.

- Blood pressure is high i.e. 140 or more for the systolic and 90 or more for the diastolic

- Fasting insulin level is more than 5 µIU(micro international units per milliliter)

- You gain weight with a lot of ease and cannot find a solution on how to stop or lose it.

- BMI (Body mass index) is in excess of 25. To determine your BMI, divide your weight in kilograms against height in square meters (m²).

- You have low triglycerides i.e. low good HDL cholesterol

- Your waist from the belly button measures 40 inches (101.6 cm) for men and 35 inches (88.9 cm) or more for ladies.

- You feel cranky or fatigued when you skip a meal or when you go hungry

- You crave for junk food to calm you down

- You feel anxious, irritable, and shaky after going for more than three hours without eating.

- You suffer from Polycystic Ovary Syndrome (PCOS), which is a condition that is characterized by cysts on the ovaries, irregular periods, acne, increased growth of hair, and /or sometimes infertility

How To Reset Insulin

To reset insulin, you have to do the following:

Reduce The Amount Of Carbs From Your Diet

Carbs are the ones that raise insulin and blood sugar levels the most when compared to the other three major macronutrients (carbs, protein and fat). This is the reason why you will want to cut back on carb rich foods. If you really want to lose weight, then a low carb diet could be the best course of action.

Watch The Amount Of Food You Eat

Human beings tend to overeat every now and then but this is a habit worth discouraging. While the pancreas secretes different amounts of insulin depending on the amount and type of food you consume, downing a hefty portion in one sitting can cause **hyper-insulinemia**. This is when you have high levels of insulin in your body. This is true especially if you are an overweight person with insulin resistance.

In one study for instance, some obese individuals struggling with insulin resistance who were made to eat a 1,300-calorie meal were found to have **double** the amount of insulin as people with normal weight who had the same meal. In contrast, consuming a smaller quantity of calories has time after time shown to decrease insulin levels and improve insulin sensitivity among obese or overweight people despite the food they eat.

Eliminate Sugar

Did you know that you can to reset your insulin pathway within a couple of days? All you need to do is to eliminate all sugar and sugar related products or substitutes from your diet. You know all the usual suspects here: soda, muffins, doughnuts, cookies and all the sugar substitutes as well (apart from **Stevia**).

Keep away from the following sugary substances: maple syrup, molasses, splenda (sucralose), agave, brown sugar, honey, and white table sugar. Many other substances we consume also contain hidden sugars. Such products include: sauces, packaged cereals, salad dressings and ketchup.

The American Heart Association (AHA) recommends 25 grams of sugar per day but in this case, you will only be taking 15 grams per day, 10 grams less to reset insulin. The next time you go out shopping, inspect product labels and look out for the grams of sugar on each label. This will enable you to choose products that contain little amounts of sugar.

Use Cinnamon

Cinnamon is a delicious and sweet smelling spice and it is packed with health boosting antioxidants. Studies show that healthy people and patients with insulin resistance who use this spice can improve insulin sensitivity and decrease insulin levels.

In a study, young people who consumed liquids with a lot of sugar in them were still able to manage having lower insulin levels after using cinnamon for the entire 2 weeks than when they drank the sugary liquids and taking a placebo.

In a another study, healthy persons who eat rice pudding with 1 and a half teaspoons of cinnamon in it had considerably lower insulin responses than people who had eaten rice pudding without cinnamon.

Engage In Physical Activity

Regular exercise not only helps to burn calories but it can also prevent you from developing resistance to insulin. If you are already insulin resistant, exercise could help you regain your insulin sensitivity.

A study published in the open access journal PLoS Biology in August 2010 showed how exercise increased IL-6 and IL-10 protein levels in the hypothalamus of the overweight rats. It was also discovered that both IL-6 and IL-10 molecules increase the sensitivity of both leptin and insulin.

You can try doing low intensity exercises like walking, jogging, cycling, dancing, swimming, skipping rope, sport and even doing some household chores. 20 to 30 minutes of physical activity per day is enough to up your fitness levels. There are plenty of activities that you can do to increase your heart rate. If you are not very physically fit, you can start slowly and then work your way up gradually as you increase the frequency and intensity.

Keep Away From Refined Carbohydrates

The world around us moves fast and we have to play catch up so much so that we have no time to prepare a nice home cooked meal using fresh food. We eat refined foods while on the go because they require little or no preparation time. But this shouldn't be the case since consuming such foods, and especially those with refined carbohydrates regularly bring with them a number of health hazards. High insulin levels and obesity are just some of those problems.

Refined carbohydrates for instance are said to have a high **glycemic index** (GI). This is the scale that determines the ability of a particular type of food to elevate the levels of blood sugar. The glycemic load takes into account the quantity of digestible carbs present in one serving as well as the glycemic index.

Researchers have been conducting studies to compare the different types of foods containing different glycemic loads to establish whether they have varying effects on the insulin levels. Eating a food that is high on glycemic load was found to spike insulin levels way much more than consuming the same amount of food with a low glycemic load even when the carbohydrate contents of both the two foods are equal. Thus, it is important to swap refined carbs that are digested and absorbed quicker with those that are digested a bit slower as this may help lower insulin levels.

Examples of such foods are: broccoli, carrots, doongora and basmati rice, brown rice, long grain, rye and whole grain bread, bircher muesli, oats, bran, sourdough bread, buckwheat, couscous, pasta, yams, corn, sweet potatoes, barley, quinoa, almond milk, soy milk, lentils and kiwi, Nicola and Carisma potato varieties, zucchini, cauliflower, rice noodles, soba noodles, semolina, freekeh, beans, peas and celery.

Consume Soluble Fiber

Soluble fiber dissolves in water to form a gel-like mixture that slows down food movement through the digestive tract. Soluble fiber is found in oats, hazelnuts, sunflower seeds, flaxseeds, guavas, apples, carrots, apricots, nectarines, figs kidney beans, turnips, broccoli, sweet potatoes, avocadoes, Brussels sprouts, lima beans and black beans among others.

According to an observational study, filling up on soluble fiber leaves you feeling satiated. It also keeps the blood sugar, cholesterol and insulin in check after a meal. In addition, friendly bacteria in your guts feed off soluble fiber. In turn, they decrease insulin resistance and improve your overall gut health. In the same study, women who consumed the largest amount of soluble fiber had a 50% less chance of developing insulin resistance as compared to women who had the smallest amount of soluble fiber

Eat The Right Amount And Type Of Protein

Consuming enough protein every day could help you control insulin levels as well as your weight. Excessive protein consumption however can sometimes increase the secretion of insulin so that your muscles can absorb amino acids.

In addition, some proteins stimulate greater insulin response than others. For instance, whey and casein proteins that are both found in dairy products can raise insulin levels a lot more even than bread does when consumed by healthy people.

The best types of proteins to consume if you want to reset insulin resistance are those from fatty fish such as mackerel, herring, anchovies, salmon and sardines. Apart from providing you with high quality protein, they are also the best sources of long chain omega-3 fatty acids you will find around.

There is even evidence to show that fatty fish can help bring down insulin resistance especially if you are suffering from PCOS (polycystic ovary syndrome), obesity or gestational diabetes. In one study, a female patient suffering from PCOS recorded a remarkable 8.4% decrease in insulin levels after she took fish oil. In another study, some obese children and adolescents took fish supplements and after tests, they were found to have significantly low levels of triglycerides (bad cholesterol) and insulin resistance.

… Hormone Reset Diet Meal Plan

How To Reset Estrogen Dominance

Self-Assessment

You need to reset estrogen if you meet at least 4 of the criteria below:

- Difficulty in losing weight and gaining weight rapidly ✓ especially in the butt and hips
- You've been diagnosed with rosacea - a skin condition that causes visible blood vessels or redness in your face (which is usually triggered by dairy, spicy foods, red wine, skin products or heat)
- Frequent headaches or migraines
- Gallbladder problems
- Bloating problems ✓
- Low sex drive ✓
- Brain fog and memory loss
- Hair loss
- Insomnia

- Bloating problems i.e. Water retention

- Breast tenderness or swelling

- Cold hands and feet

- Dry skin and edema

- Increased size of bra cup or non-cancerous breast lumps

- Pain or discomfort in the LV3 (i.e. the concave area located between your second toe and the big toe somewhere on top of your foot especially when you massage the area) which is a symptom of estrogen dominance and a sign of liver stagnation.

- Painful periods, fibroids, endometriosis, heavy bleeding, postmenopausal bleeding or abnormal pap smears

- Autoimmune abnormalities (when your own immune system launches an attack on your body tissues) such as Thyroiditis (Hashimoto's disease).

- Depression, irritability, anxiety, mini breakdowns (over the most ridiculous things), mood swings, etc.

How To Reset Estrogen

To reset estrogen dominance, you need to do the following:

Hormone Reset Diet Meal Plan

Keep Off Alcohol *Don't Drink much now*

Alcohol is one of the leading causes of increased levels of estrogen in the bloodstream even though some wines such as the Spanish and Sardinian wines are rich in antioxidants that may help flush out estrogen. In addition, alcohol may amplify some effects of low testosterone. Since alcohol contains a lot of calories, it could lead to weight gain.

Meat And Dairy

Many animal products contain traces of estrogen including milk. As a matter of fact, it is not only the beef cattle that are fed with estrogen, but also the dairy animals. Cows are given high doses of estrogen to increase the amount of milk they produce. When you consume such dairy products, your estrogen levels increase.

Moreover, consuming red meat increases estrogen and affects your estrobolome. This is the part of your microbiome (the microbes that dwell in your gut and their DNA) that manages estrogen levels.

Desist From Hormonal Birth Control

If possible, you need to discontinue with these hormonal birth control methods if you have been using them because it messes with your hormonal balance. Apart from hormonal contraceptives, there are other medications that could increase estrogen. These include phenothiazines (used to treat emotional and mental disorders) and some antibiotics.

Beauty And Personal Care Products

Beauty and personal care products are some of the most notorious culprits for introducing xenoestrogens into your body. Lipstick for instance contains some toxic metals such as lead. It is said that the average woman swallows about 10 pounds of lipstick in her lifetime. If you must wear lipstick or any other make-up for that matter, make sure it is totally organic.

Some Legumes

A number of legumes such as soy, peanuts and lentils are good for your health in many ways. For instance, they can be a good meat substitute because of the relatively high amounts of protein they provide. However, such legumes contain phytoestrogens and if consumed in large amounts, such legumes could increase your estrogen level considerably. Phytoestrogens are compounds that occur naturally in plants. They have a similar chemical structure to your own body's estrogen. When consumed, phytoestrogens may affect you in the same way as estrogen produced by your body since they bind to the same receptors that your own estrogen does.

Legumes reduce the risk of metabolic syndrome and may support your heart health. Rather than eliminating them from your diet, you should consider consuming a few servings once or twice a week.

Some Grains

Some grains contain a fungus known as **zearalenone,** which has been shown to increase the level of estrogen. Some scientists from Europe studied the fungus and found that 32% of over 5,000 mixed cereal and grain samples were contaminated with the fungus.

However, there is no way to determine whether a product is contaminated or free from zearalenone. If you are looking to avoid ingesting the fungus, then you ought to limit your intake of grains such as maize, rice, wheat or barley.

There are certain foods that may be able to reduce the level of estrogen in your blood. Based on the conclusions of these studies, the following are the foods that may help lower estrogen.

Turmeric And Curcumin

Turmeric contains a chemical known as curcumin. A study in 2013 showed that curcumin may help decrease estrogen levels. However, the scientists noted that this result was achieved in cells outside the body and they are unsure whether curcumin may have the same effect inside the human body. Yet still, another study published in 2014 showed how huge doses of curcumin were able to increase the levels of testosterone in rats.

Mushrooms

Researchers have revealed that certain varieties of mushrooms such as the Portobello and the white button could lower your estrogen levels while increasing your testosterone levels.

Cruciferous Veggies

Cruciferous veggies such as cabbages, broccoli, bok choy and cauliflower contain isoflavones. Several studies were conducted and it was suggested that these isoflavones may prevent your body from converting testosterone to estrogen. These vegetables also contain sulforaphane, which according to studies, can help restore estrogen receptor expression. In addition, vegetables from the Brassicae family contain the Indole-3-carbinol compound, which has been found to be a negative regulator of estrogen.

Soy Products

As stated earlier, soy and its products such as tofu and Edamame contain phytoestrogens. Initial studies raised fears within some sectors that phytoestrogens could increase levels of estrogen in the blood. However, they could have the opposite effect. Later on, research suggested that the plant based estrogens do not affect the levels of estrogen in human bodies.

Phytoestrogens are 'weaker' than estrogen that is produced by your body. When phytoestrogens make their way into your body cells, they push out your own estrogen. This way, eating more phytoestrogens could reduce your won estrogen level. In addition, phytoestrogens may help reduce the risk of developing estrogen related diseases such as prostate cancer.

Estrogen Dominance Reset Supplements

The following is a list of some supplements that you may find useful in your quest to ending estrogen dominance: folate, vitamin B12 and B6, maca, omega-3 fatty acids,

Passionflower, Di-indoly-lmethane (DIM), alpha lipoic acid and milk thistle. Use these as prescribed by your pharmacist.

In addition, it is worth remembering that estrogen is secreted by the bowel. If stool remains in the bowel, then estrogen is reabsorbed. This is why you need to get enough **fiber** as well.

How To Reset Thyroid

Self-Assessment

You need to reset your thyroid if you meet at least 4 of the criteria below:

- Thyroid antibodies commonly known as Hashimoto's disease or autoimmune Thyroiditis or any other autoimmune condition

- A first or second degree celiac disease

- Chronic acne or eczema, unexplained skin rashes and hair loss

- Attention deficit, autism, short stature, low birth weight when you were born (less than 5 pounds)

- Menstrual disorders, unexplained infertility or repeated miscarriages (three or more)

- Migraines and headaches

- Mineral and/or vitamin deficiencies such as iron deficient anaemia

- Difficulty in losing weight (stubborn fat) and gaining weight rapidly

- Walking with a wide gait, difficulty walking or a loss of coordination and balance

- Chronic fatigue and brain fog

- Schizophrenia, depression or anxiety

- Restless legs syndrome

- Bone pain, joint aches

- Acid reflux, Diagnosis of irritable bowel disease (GERD), diarrhea and constipation, food poisoning, frequent or smelly gas, recurring abdominal bloating or pain

How To Reset The Thyroid

To improve thyroid functioning, you need to do the following:

Eliminate Gluten

Gluten is a type of protein found in grains. Gluten is the main food group where substantive proof supports a connection to an autoimmune disease of the thyroid that holds back your metabolism. Studies show that people who live with

Hashimoto's disease, which is the main cause of hypothyroidism, could also develop celiac disease, another autoimmune disease in which your body mistakenly attacks and causes damage to the gut area. This happens especially when you eat gluten.

Eliminate all foods made from grain including flour. Avoid foods such as kamut, rice, millet, spelt, durum, corn, oats, barley, rye and wheat and any other byproducts made from any of these grains

Also eliminate all processed foods that contain grain, thickeners or gluten derivatives. Such include all spices, beer, cream sauces, pasta, bread, pizza, processed cheeses, nondairy creamers, dried soup mixes, canned soups, salad dressings, ice cream, pickles, mustard, luncheon meats and hot dogs.

As a substitute for grains, you can eat kelp noodles, baked sweet potatoes, coconut flour, romaine lettuce, dehydrated vegetable crackers, flaxseed crackers, yams, roasted seaweed and coconut wraps.

Avoid Or Limit Foods With Goitrogens

Goitrogens are naturally occurring compounds that affect thyroid health by inhibiting the synthesis of thyroid hormones. The word 'Goitrogens' comes from the word 'goiter' which basically means enlargement of the thyroid gland. If your thyroid is having trouble in producing the thyroid hormone, it usually swells as a way to compensate for its inadequate production of the thyroid hormone. Goitrogens also limit the amount of iodine that your body can take in.

Normally, foods with Goitrogens in them don't cause many problems to many of the people with thyroid problems. To be on the safe side, it is possible to limit the amount of Goitrogens you consume by sautéing or steaming them. Doing this limits the active goitrogenic compounds by up to a third. It is therefore not advisable to consume such foods raw and limit these to 6 or 8 servings per week.

Examples of foods that are high in Goitrogens include: soy, turnips, rutabagas, radishes, mustard and mustard greens, kohlrabi, kale, cauliflower cabbage, Brussel sprouts, collard greens broccoli and bok choy. Basically, all cruciferous vegetables contain Goitrogens. Others foods include peanuts, pine nuts, millet, strawberries, peaches, cassava, sweet potatoes, Edamame, tempeh and tofu.

Don't get this wrong. These are nutritious foods and their benefits far outweigh their downsides. To offset the effects of

Goitrogens in them, accompany them with foods that are high in iodine.

Be Wary Of Extremely Low Carb And Low Calorie Diets

We cannot deny that indeed low carb diets are very effective if you want to lose weight. But did you know that low carb diets could potentially worsen fatigue in people suffering from hypothyroidism?

While that doesn't necessarily mean that you avoid such diets altogether, but perhaps you should start a low carb diet if you do it moderately. For example, consuming 20% or 30% of calories from carbs would be a good place to start. Only after your thyroid conversion and function has been optimized can you consider decreasing the carb intake further.

Likewise, diets that restrict caloric intake could make the functioning of your thyroid worse. When you restrict calories, your body could interpret that as a sign that you are starving. In order to preserve energy, the production of reverse T3 is increased and the subsequent conversion of T4 to T3 is decreased.

The following are some of the minerals you need that are vital for optimal thyroid health:

Zinc

Zinc has a way of 'activating' thyroid hormones so that they are used by the body according to studies. Moreover, zinc helps the body to regulate TSH, which is the hormone that signals the thyroid gland to release thyroid hormones.

However, there are little or no reported cases of zinc deficiencies in the developed countries because zinc is fortified in the food supplies. If you suffer from hypothyroidism, you should consume more zinc rich foods such as: kidney beans, lima beans, eggs, Swiss cheese, cocoa powder, oats, pumpkin seeds, flax seeds, sesame seeds and oysters.

Other sources are spinach, mushrooms, turkey, chicken, brown rice, yogurt, garlic, cashews, peas, chickpeas, crab, shellfish, almonds, lamb and peanuts.

Selenium

Selenium, like zinc, has a way of helping the body to 'activate' thyroid hormones too. Selenium has antioxidant properties.

This means that it may prevent free radicals from damaging the thyroid gland.

It is not advisable to take selenium supplements unless prescribes by the doctor. The reason being that supplements usually provide large doses and studies show that selenium could intoxicate the body if taken in large amounts.

There are plenty of foods that would nourish your body with this essential mineral. These include: shrimp, chia seeds, swordfish, liverwurst, mackerel, pork chop, whelk, whole wheat pasta, lobster, cuttlefish, kidney, liver, anchovies, octopus, salmon, sunflower seeds, mussels, yellowfin, tuna, oysters, mustard seeds, asparagus, mushrooms, cod, sardines, soya beans and brazil nuts.

Iodine

Iodine is one of the most essential minerals because the thyroid needs it to synthesize thyroid hormones. This is why people who are iodine deficient are at risk of developing hypothyroidism. Sadly, iodine deficiency is very common and affects almost one third of the people on the globe. It is not so common however in developed countries because table is usually iodized.

Apart from iodized salt, any iodine deficiency can also be rectified by eating foods such as sea weeds/vegetables such as hiziki, wakame kelp, kombu kelp, arame kelp and nori. Other foods include chocolate, creamed corn, prunes, eggs, albacore tuna, salmon, snapper, cod, organic potatoes, lima beans, raw organic cheese, yogurt, raw milk, Cape Cod cranberries, eggs and Himalayan pink salt

How To Reset Testosterone

Self-Assessment

You need to reset your testosterone if you meet at least 4 of the criteria below:

- Feeling irritable or shaky when you haven't eaten sugar or refined carbs

- Itchy eyes with bags or dark circles under the eyes or even mucus in the eyes after waking up

- Weight gain

- Lower sex drive

- Irritability, depression, anxiety and mood swings

- Bronchitis or chest congestion and colds

- Reduced muscle mass and strength

- Burping, heartburn, nausea, gas in the tummy and bloating

- Rashes, dry skin, or hives, itching ears or tinnitus

- Brain fog and poor memory

- Puffy looking face caused by water retention

- Worsening bad breath

- Achy joints

How To Reset Testosterone

To improve testosterone functioning, you need to do the following:

Avoid Drug, Alcohol And Substance Abuse

Abusing alcohol and drugs brings about lower testosterone. This is according to the National Institute of Alcohol Abuse and Alcoholism (NIAAA). Men who drank moderate amounts of booze every day for 21 days experienced a 7% decrease in testosterone. It is ok therefore to limit your drinking to a glass or two of wine or beer to avoid a significant drop in testosterone levels.

Avoid Stressors

You should try and get away from repetitive stressors in your life. Elevated stress levels increase the production of the hormone cortisol. According to a study conducted in 2016, elevated cortisol levels brought about by stressful events can have a negative impact on your testosterone. These hormones work in a see-saw manner; if one shoots up, the other one goes down.

Unnatural increase in cortisol and stress could also increase the amount of food you consume. And this causes weight gain and storage of harmful body fat and eventually your testosterone levels are negatively impacted.

Get Enough Sleep

Inadequate sleep could adversely affect your health and could greatly impact your testosterone negatively. While the ideal amount of sleep may vary from one person to another, studies show that if you sleep for only 5 hours one night, you could have a reduction of around 15% of your testosterone levels.

Those who sleep for only 4 hours per night could have borderline deficient levels. For every extra hour of sleep you get, testosterone levels could improve by 15% in average. Research shows that you should get about 7 to 8 hours of uninterrupted sleep per night for optimum long term health and normal testosterone levels.

Expose Yourself To Some Sunshine

It is important to get at least 15 minutes of direct sunshine every day. Vitamin D is a natural testosterone booster but despite its importance, people spend their time inside their offices leading to a deficiency in this essential vitamin. Luckily, there are vitamin D supplements in drug stores.

A 2011 study that was conducted for 12 months found that supplementing with 3,300 UI of Vitamin D3 every day improved testosterone levels by approximately 25%. In the elderly generation for instance, calcium and vitamin D optimized testosterone levels. This reduced their chances of falling. Other than supplements, foods such as cereal, dairy products and fatty fishes are all excellent sources of vitamin D.

Herbal Testosterone Boosters

The herb that is most researched as far as testosterone is concerned is ashwagandha. Studies show that the herb has powerful effects on reproductive health and testosterone levels. It increased testosterone levels in infertile men to around 17%. In addition, ashwagandha has also been shown to decrease levels of cortisol (stress hormone) by 30% on average.

Ginger is also another testosterone boosting herb. According to a study conducted in 2012, a group of people took ginger supplement for 3 months. Their testosterone increased by 17.7%

Plastic-Packaged Or Canned Foods

Food and beverage that are packaged in plastic or canned can take a toll on your hormones. For instance, drinking water from some plastic bottles or reheating food in plastic containers may release chemicals such as bisphenol S and bisphenol A (BPA).

A study conducted in 2013 shows that men who work in factories with high BPA levels had lower levels of testosterone and androstenedione (a hormone that converts testosterone into estrogen).

Processed Foods

Most prepackaged and frozen foods and snacks are usually processed. They offer you little or no nutritional value whatsoever. In addition, they normally contain plenty of sugar, fat and salt. Processed foods contain excessive amounts of Trans fats. According to a study conducted in

2017, these trans fats could reduce or impair testosterone functioning.

How To Reset Your Growth Hormone

Self-Assessment

You need to reset your Growth Hormone if you meet at least 4 of the criteria below:

- Frequent skin reactions such as hives, red skin, itchy bumps, rash etc.

- Sinus infection (a tendency towards sinusitis)

- Bloating or an Irritable bowel

- Addiction to cheese or milk-based treats such as latte or frappuccino; an unsettling feeling when such aren't available

- Swelling of the throat, mouth, tongue, face and lips

- Anaphylaxis - a severe and allergic reaction that causes swelling which can make it difficult for you to either talk, swallow or breathe

- Sneezing, wheezing, coughing, itchy, gurgling belly, and watery eyes, stuffy or runny nose especially after eating dairy.

How To Reset Your Growth Hormone

To help optimize your Human Growth Hormone levels, you need to do the following:

Supplement With Gamma Aminobutyric Acid (GABA)

GABA is a non-protein amino acid neurotransmitter that facilitates communication among your brain cells. It is a well known calming agent for your nervous system and your brain and is often prescribed to insomniac patients. Interestingly, GABA can also be used to boost your HGH levels.

Studies show that supplementing with GABA could increase HGH production by 200% after exercising and a400% increment at rest. Additionally, taking GABA supplements could also further increase HGH production since it improves the quality of sleep given the fact that night time secretion of HGH is linked to sleep quality and depth. However, the only downside was that most of the studies conducted discovered that many of these GABA supplemented HGH increases worked for the short-term. As such, GABAs long lasting advantages for human growth hormone still remain uncertain.

Avoid Eating Just Before Bedtime

The human body usually releases plenty of HGH especially during the night. Because many foods result in increased insulin production, experts suggest that you avoid eating just before you got to bed. The foods you ought to avoid in particular are those that are high in protein and carbs. These could spike your insulin levels and this could eventually prevent some of the HGH from being released. Just remember that insulin levels plummet after 2 or 3 hours when you're done eating. Therefore, eat more than 3 hours before your bedtime.

Cut Back On Refined Carbs And Sugar Consumption

Increased insulin levels have been found to reduce the production of Growth Hormone. There are two culprits in particular, sugar and refined carbohydrates, and if you were to limit your consumption, that would go a long way in optimizing your growth hormone levels.

In one study, it was discovered that people suffering from diabetes had 3 or 4 times lower the amount of HGH as opposed to the healthy people. Apart from affecting insulin levels, excessive consumption for refined carbs and sugar is also a major factor in weight gain and obesity affects your levels of HGH.

Supplement With L-Arginine

L-Arginine, also arginine is an amino acid that helps your body to synthesize proteins. Even when taken on its own, arginine can boost HGH levels. Even though most people tend to use it alongside workout regimen, studies show little increase in HGH after the exercises.

However, studies show that if taken on its own without any workout regimen, arginine could significantly increase the production of HGH. In addition, another study also examined which dosage would yield better HGH results between 45 mg per pound (100 mg per kg) of body weight or 114 mg per pound (250 mg per kg) of body weight. For the lower dose, there was no little or no effect. However, those who took the higher dosage recorded a 60% increment in HGH when they were asleep.

Try Intermittent Fasting

Multiple studies thus far have shown that fasting can significantly increase the production of HGH. One study in particular found that just three days into a fast, HGH production increased by more than 300%. After fasting for seven days, HGH had now increased by a whopping 1,250%. Many other studies have had similar results with most of them doubling or tripling the levels of HGH after just 2 or 3 days of fasting.

However, fasting for days does not mean fasting continuously a day after the other since it is not sustainable in the long term. Intermittent fasting however is more sustainable. This is because you deliberately choose to skip a particular meal or meals for a set period of time such that you alternate between periods of fasting and eating.

Intermittent fasting helps you optimize your HGH levels in two major ways. First, it keeps the levels of insulin very low for as long as you are in the fasted state, since insulin is secreted after you have eaten. And research shows that an increase in insulin could disrupt the natural production of your growth hormones.

Secondly, intermittent fasting is a proven and efficient method of hacking away stubborn fat. Decreased body fat directly translates into increased production of growth hormone according to studies.

There are multiple methods of intermittent fasting available and each is tailored to suit your lifestyle or preference:

a) **Eat stop eat** - which involves fasting for at least 2 alternate days each week i.e. a 24 hour fast once or twice per week.

b) **The warrior diet** - is a 20 hour fast followed by a 4 hours eating window. This basically means fasting for the entire day and then eating to your fill within the 4 hour window.

c) **Alternate day fasting** - you are required to alternate between one day of eating and then eating very little on the next day (fasting every other day).

d) **The Leangains protocol** - you are required to fast for 16 hours and break the fast for the remaining 8 hour window of the day

e) **The 5:2 fast diet** - involves normal dieting for 5 days (of your choice) of the week and then proceeding to restrict your calorie intake for the rest of the 2 days.

Try The Sauna

A sauna, also known as a sudatory, is a small building or room that is designed for use by people to experience dry or wet heat to induce sweating. Sitting in the sauna is a form of hyper-thermic conditioning and it does result into a sustained and massive release of growth hormones. The level of HGH increment depends on the temperature and the time you spend sitting on the sauna. Thus the longer and hooter the session is, the more growth hormone you liberate.

According to studies, the relevant results were as follows:

- Two 20 minute sessions done at a temperature of 176° F (80° C) increased growth hormone by 200%

- Two 15 minute sessions done at a temperature of 212° F (100° C) increased growth hormone by 500%

- Two hour sessions per day for 3 days at a temperature of 176° F (80° C) increased HGH 16 times over.

N.B: to prevent dehydration or a severe heat stroke, DO NOT overdo the sauna. Listen to the limits of your body. More is not always better.

With everything we've learned so far in mind, now is time to put it all into action by following a 21 day plan that will see your body bouncing into a fat burning mode in no time! Let's focus on hormone reset diet recipes next.

Hormone Reset Recipes

Shakes And Smoothies

Berry And Coconut Smoothie

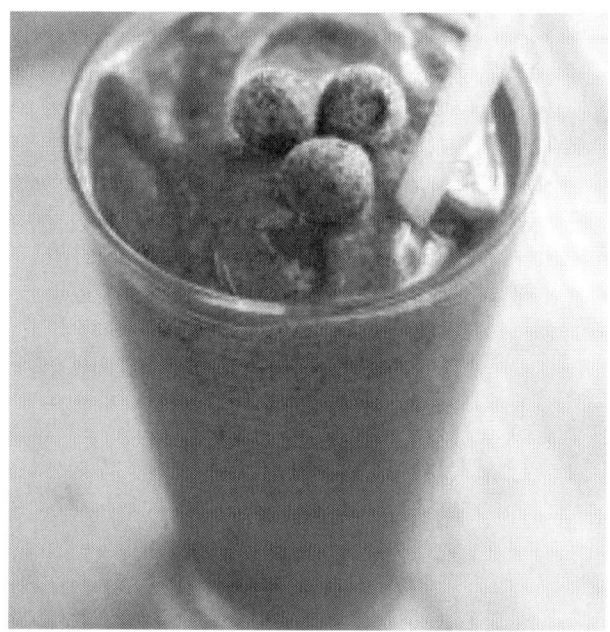

Serves 1

Ingredients

1 scoop collagen protein powder

1 tablespoon pure maple syrup or raw honey

1 cup full-fat unsweetened coconut milk

1 teaspoon maca powder

1 handful dark leafy greens of your choice

1 cup frozen mixed berries

Directions

Put all the ingredients in a high powered blender and blend until smooth then serve.

Vanilla Green Milkshake

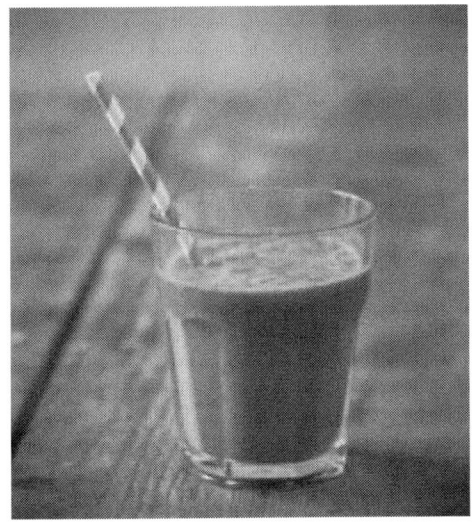

Serves 1

Ingredients

4 or 6 pieces of dinosaur kale without stems

½ avocado

2 scoops vanilla shake

1 or 2 tablespoons chia seeds soaked in unsweetened hemp, almond or coconut milk for 3 to 4 hours

Handful of ice cubes

Additional unsweetened hemp, almond or coconut milk to achieve your desired consistency and taste

Directions

Put all the ingredients in a high powered blender and blend until smooth then serve.

Ginger Rhubarb Cider

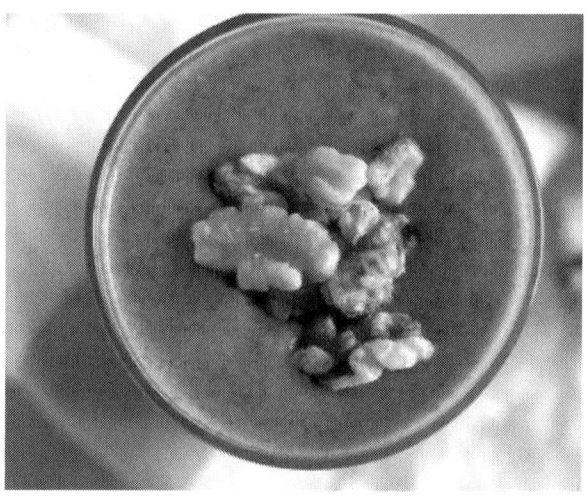

Hormone Reset Diet Meal Plan

Makes 2 servings

Ingredients

½ inch ginger

½ juiced lemon

1 chopped apple

1 tablespoon of apple cider vinegar

1½ ounces (3 tablespoons) Swiss chard

2 ounces rhubarb

3 tablespoons of walnuts for healthy fats

1 cup water

2 handfuls of ice cubes

Directions

Blend until smooth and serve.

Sweet Spirit

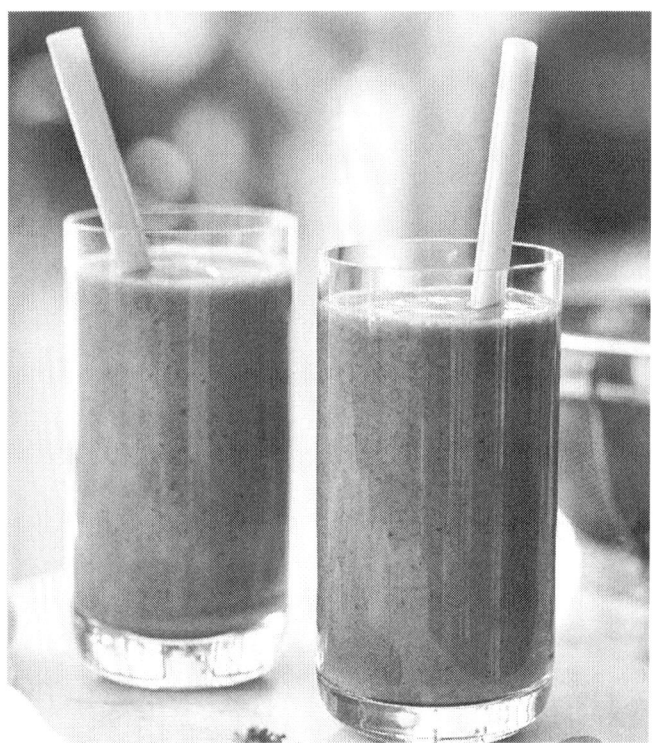

Servings: 1 – 2

Ingredients

1 scoop of hemp, vanilla, pea or pumpkin protein powder

1 tablespoon spirulina

½ cup of almond milk

½ cup of blueberries

½ frozen banana

¼ avocado

1 cup of water

Directions

Place all the ingredients in the jar and turn on the motor. Increase the speed to the maximum and let it run for more than a minute until smooth.

Kale And Sunflower Smoothie

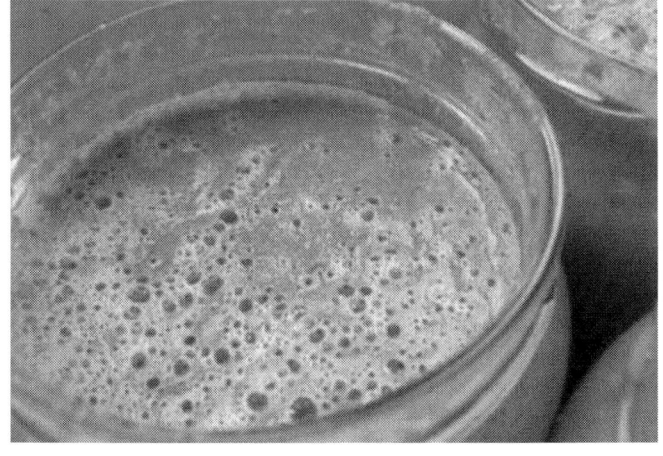

Servings: 2 – 3

Ingredients

2 tablespoons of sunflower seed butter

1½ cups of stemmed and chopped kale

1 cup of coconut water

1 frozen banana

1 peeled, cored and chopped Bartlett pear

1 tablespoon of honey (you can have more or less depending on your preference)

½ cup of cubed papaya fruit (you can use mango as an alternative)

Directions

Steam the kale by placing a steaming rack over a boiling water pot. Ensure that there is no contact between the rack and the water. Cover the kale and steam it for 5 to 10 minutes until it appears wilted. Don't put it in the blender when hot; allow it to cool slightly.

Combine the kale and all the other ingredients into your blender.

Blend at high speed for 2 or 3 minutes until it is fine then serve immediately.

Savory Shake

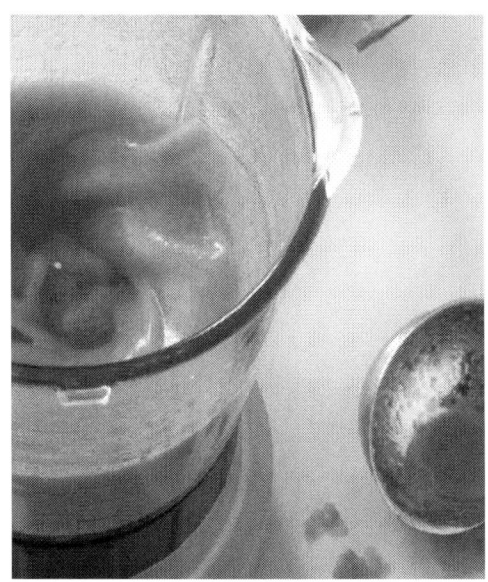

Servings: 1

Ingredients

1 to 2 scoops vanilla protein powder

½ cup unsweetened coconut milk

Warm cooked vegetables

1 tablespoon miso

1 avocado

1 cup vegetable stock, fish or chicken

Directions

Blend all the ingredients until the desired smoothness then drink up before it cools

Breakfast Recipes

Adaptogenic Tea

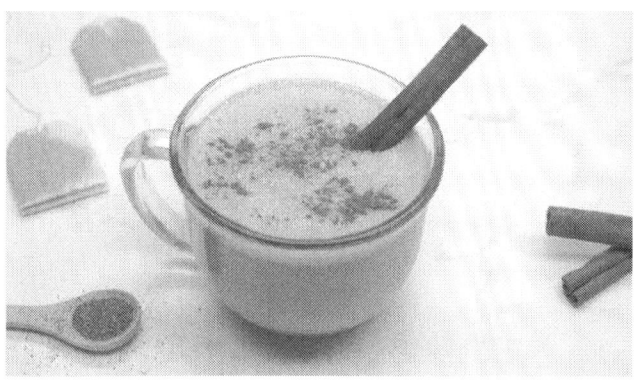

Serves 1

Ingredients

½ teaspoon pure vanilla extract

1 pinch ground cinnamon

¼ cup full-fat unsweetened coconut milk

1 cup boiled and filtered water

1 tulsi or organic holy basil tea bag

Directions

Boil water and pour it into a mug with the tea bag then steep for 7 or 10 minutes.

Stir in the coconut milk and vanilla extract.

Garnish with a pinch of ground cinnamon. Stir and enjoy.

Chocolate Dipped Banana Bites

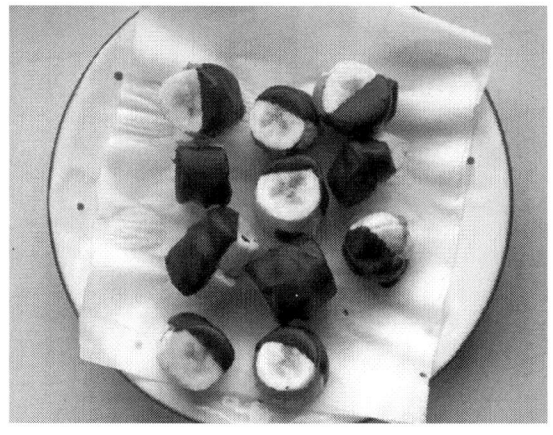

Serves 1

Ingredients

1 small skinless banana cut into 1 inch slices

2 tablespoons semi sweet chocolate chips

Directions

Pour the chocolate chips in a glass bowl.

Microwave them on high heat for 1 minute to melt.

Dip each banana piece in the molten chocolate.

Serve immediately.

Kraut And Eggs

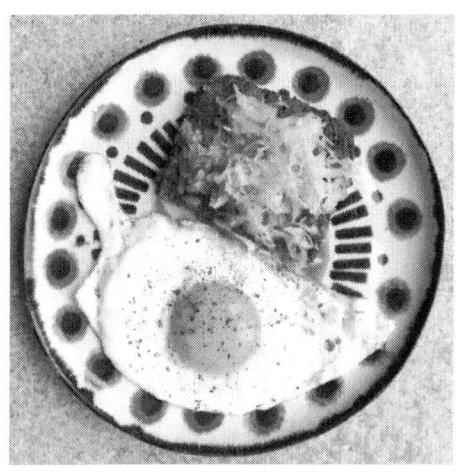

Serves 2

Ingredients

¼ or 1/2 cup sauerkraut

1 tablespoons olive or coconut oil

2 handfuls spinach

2 pastured eggs

Directions

Start by putting the olive or coconut oil to a pan over medium heat.

Whisk the eggs in a bowl.

Add spinach to the hot oil and fry until they wilt.

Add the eggs into the pan and scramble them on the spinach until they cook.

Add sauerkraut as topping then serve.

Nutty Seed Granola

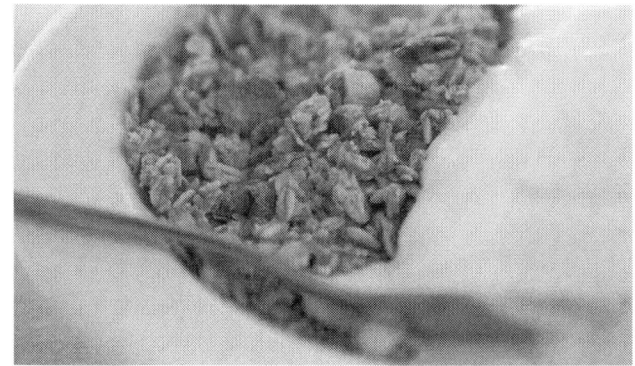

Hormone Reset Diet Meal Plan

Serves 2

Ingredients

½ teaspoon kosher salt

½ teaspoon ground cinnamon

1 teaspoon vanilla extract

3 tablespoons coconut oil

2 tablespoons water

1 teaspoon cinnamon

1 cup shredded and unsweetened coconut

½ cup flax seed / sesame seed combo

1 cup sprouted or raw pepitas (pumpkin seeds)

1 ½ cups raw almonds

1 cup raw walnuts

1 lightly beaten egg (optional - helps to make the dish crispier and holds the ingredients together)

Directions

Preheat your oven to 300° F and line a baking sheet with parchment paper.

Add the walnuts, almonds and pepitas to a food processor or blender. Pulse a couple of times to make a fine chop but don't grind them into a fine meal.

Whisk the egg white with water in a large mixing bowl until slightly foamy and bubbly.

Add the salt, cinnamon and vanilla extract to the egg white and water mixture then keep whisking.

Pour the shredded coconut and the chopped nut mixture into the mixing bowl and stir until the mixture is coated.

Spread the granola evenly on the baking sheet and let it bake for 40 minutes or until it turns crispy and golden brown.

Keep it aside and let it cool for around 10 minutes.

Using a spatula, reach under the granola to release the large clusters.

Once completely cooled, store the granola in sealable glass jar.

Serve it over dried fruit, fresh fruit or coconut yogurt.

Collagen Frappe And Tea

Serves 1

Ingredients

1 tablespoon of MCT oil

3 tablespoons of clean protein (collagen)

Brewed tea

Directions

Put all 3 ingredients in a blender and blend for half a minute or so then serve

Raw Chocolate Chia Pancakes

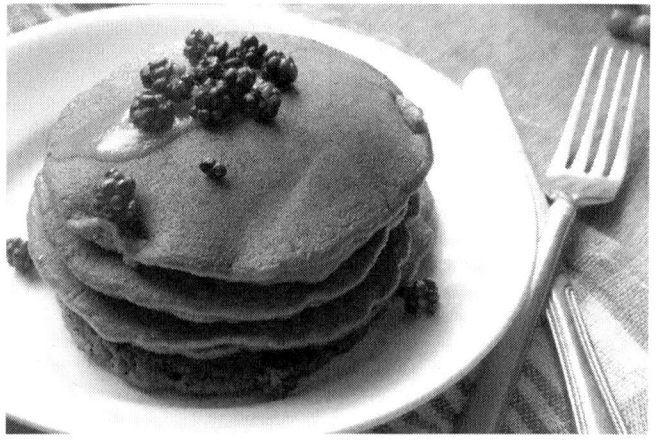

Hormone Reset Diet Meal Plan

Serves 4

Ingredients

1 teaspoon cinnamon

2 cups water

1 teaspoon maca powder

½ cup raw cacao powder

½ cup goji berries

½ cup finely ground macadamia or walnuts

1 cup chia seeds

Directions

Put all ingredients in a large bowl and mix them together.

Add water and whisk them.

Make round shapes using an ice cream scoop.

Place them on a baking tray and into the oven set at the lowest heat setting overnight. Alternatively, you can use a dehydrator set at 115 for about 7 hours.

Farmer's Wife Breakfast

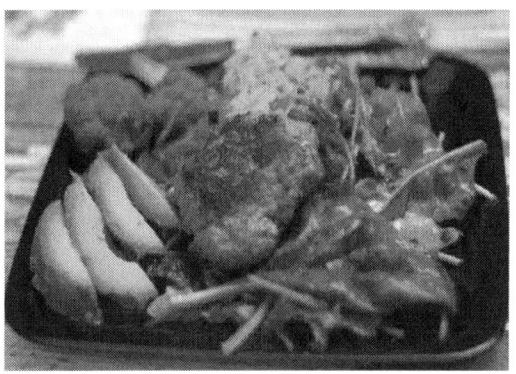

Serves 6

Ingredients for sausage

1 tablespoon of ghee

2 tablespoons coconut aminos

2 tablespoons apple cider vinegar

2 teaspoons ground fennel seed

1 teaspoon sea salt

1 pound of ground lamb (you can also use chicken or pork or a combination of any of them)

Ingredients for plate (for one)

Juice from half a lemon

Hormone Reset Diet Meal Plan

1 tablespoon olive oil

1 cup of ferments (sauerkraut and cauliflower)

Handful of organic green mix e.g. spinach, baby kale, Mizuna and arugula

½ avocado

Pinch of sea salt

Directions

Mix all sausage ingredients together, (except the ghee) and knead them well.

Shape the sausage to the shape you desire either long, flat or round.

Heat ghee in a large skillet.

Add the sausages and fry them for about 7 minutes on one side and 4 on the other.

Put the green salad mix in a separate bowl and add salt, lemon and olive until the leaves are well covered with the dressing

Serve the salad on a large plate then add the ferments, avocado and sausages on the plate.

Healthy Egg, Ham And Chips

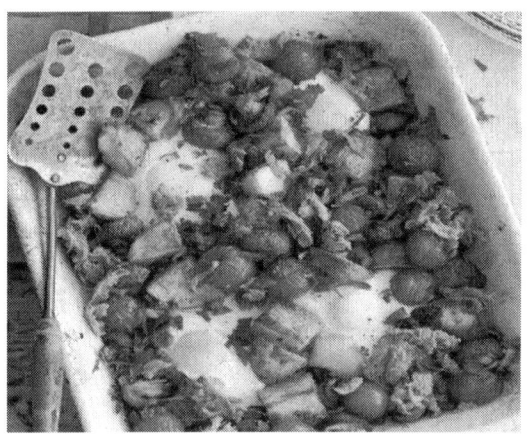

Serves 4

Ingredients

4 ounces (125 grams) pulled ham hock

4 large eggs

1 tablespoon wholegrain mustard

9 ounces (250 g) cherry tomatoes

4 fresh thyme sprigs

14 ounces (400 g) small closed cup mushrooms (halved if large)

1 tablespoon olive oil

1 roughly chopped onion

3 medium peeled potatoes and diced into ¾ inch (2 cm) cubes

Chopped fresh chives or parsley to garnish

Directions

Preheat the oven to 180° F (200° C).

Line a large non-stick roasting tin with baking parchment then throw in the onion, potato cubes, plenty of seasoning and oil. Let them roast for about 20 minutes.

Remove the tin from the oven and add the thyme and mushrooms together. Take it back to the oven for 25 more minutes or until tender and golden.

Remove from the oven again and add the mustard and cherry tomatoes. Make 4 spaces in the tin and crack the eggs in. Take it back in the oven for 8 or 10 minutes or until the egg whites are cooked.

Top with herbs and ham then serve.

Posh Beans On Toast

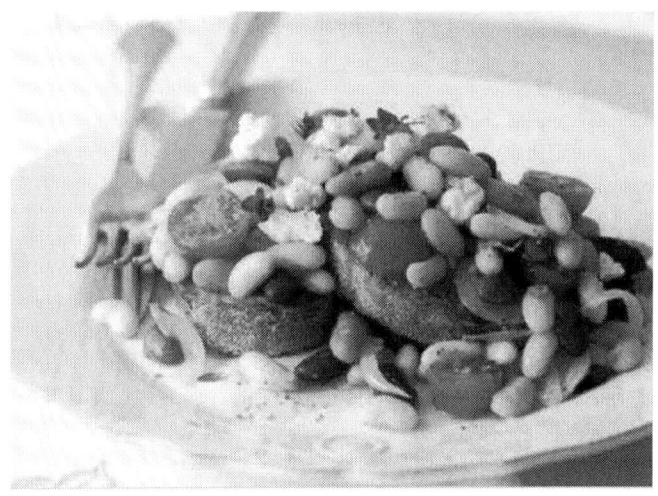

Serves 4

Ingredients

2 ounces (50 grams) vegetarian goat's cheese

8 slices crusty bread

A few sprigs of lemon thyme with leaves removed

4 ounces (125 grams) hot vegetable stock

2 tablespoons sweet chili sauce e.g. Wing Yip

5 ounces (150 g) halved cherry tomatoes

1 × 400 g can of drained cannellini beans

1 × 400 g can of drained mixed beans

¼ finely chopped chili

2 thinly sliced shallots

2 tablespoons olive oil

Directions

In a large pan, heat oil and fry the chili and shallots for 2 minutes.

Add the chili sauce, tomatoes, most of the thyme and the stock then heat for a few more minutes until the tomatoes start to cook down.

In the meantime, toast the bread and spoon the beans to the toast.

Crumble over the remaining thyme and the goat's cheese then serve immediately.

Lunch Recipes

Garlic And Basil Rice

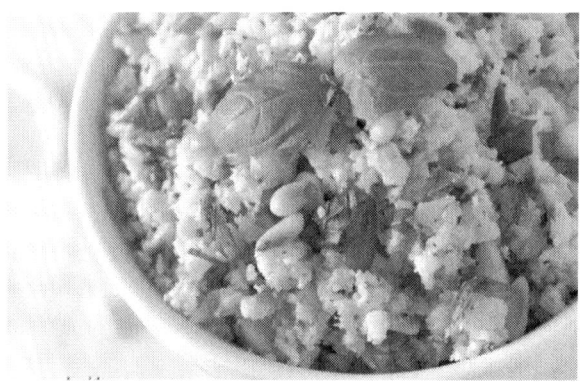

Serves 4

Ingredients

¾ cup chopped basil

3 minced shallots

1 teaspoon coconut oil

1 teaspoon fine grain sea salt

3 cloves garlic

2 tablespoons olive oil

2 full cauliflower heads

Pinch of black pepper

Additional pepper and salt to taste

Directions

Add the cauliflower florets to a food processor and pulse it until it resembles rice.

Add olive oil into a large saucepan and preheat it. Add the shallots and cook them for 5 minutes.

Add garlic and cook for 2 more minutes.

Add the cauliflower 'rice' and keep cooking until tender then add the basil for a few minutes then serve while hot.

Roasted Beets And Greens Gluten Free Pasta

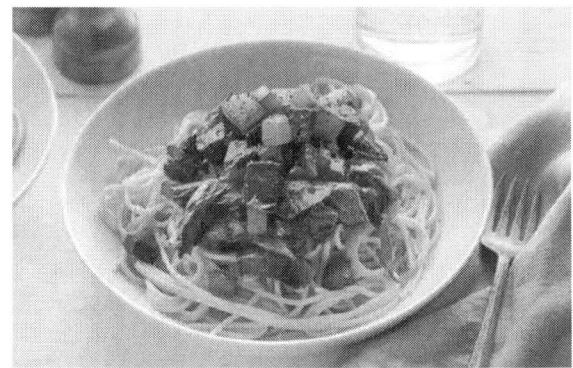

Serves 2 to 3

Ingredients

1 package gluten free pasta

2 bunches of beets with tops

1 clove garlic (crushed with garlic press)

2 tablespoons coconut oil

Freshly ground black pepper

Sea salt to taste

Directions

Cut the tops from the beets and set aside.

Wash the beets and coat them lightly with coconut oil, pepper and salt.

Preheat the oven to 435° F then roast the beets for about 45 to 50 minutes or until they get tender. Smaller pieces may only need 25 minutes and thus you need to check on them frequently.

Prepare pasta in a large saucepot as the label directs. Cook it to al dente (without overcooking since gluten free pasta can become mushy).

Remove ¾ cup pasta cooking water and reserve. Drain the pasta and return the saucepot.

Chop the beet stems and greens coarsely and set the greens aside.

Remove the beets from the oven when they're cooked and allow them to cool down a bit before slicing them into small cubes. You are also free to peel them at this stage if you so wish.

Heat oil and garlic in a nonstick 12 inch skillet over medium heat for 2 or 3 minutes until the garlic turns slightly golden. Increase the heat to medium high and add the beet greens to the skillet. Cook for 3 minutes as you stir occasionally.

Add the roasted beets and 1 teaspoon of salt then let it cook for 1 or 2 minutes or until the beet greens are wilted.

Add the reserved pasta water to the mixture a ¼ at a time until the sauce acquires the consistency you desire.

Toss well, season with pepper and salt to taste then serve over warm pasta

Lemon Chicken With Crockpot Coconut

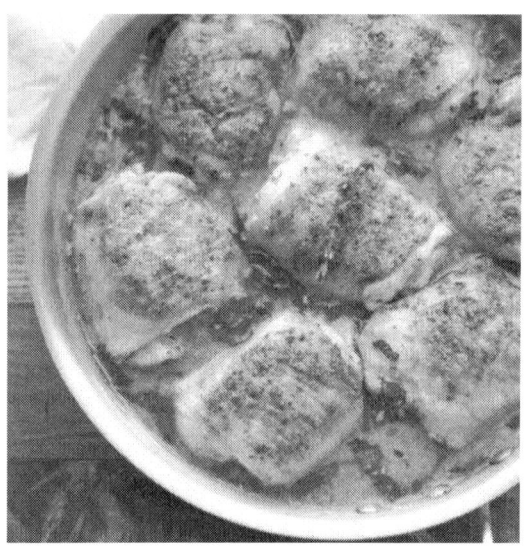

Serves 4

Ingredients

1 pinch ground black pepper

2 minced cloves of garlic

1 diced small yellow onion

½ teaspoon sea salt

½ teaspoon ground turmeric

1 tablespoon curry powder

Juice from one lemon

1 can full fat coconut milk

4 chicken breasts

Directions

Begin by whisking together the seasoning and the coconut milk (with its cream).

Add the chicken breasts to the base of a Crockpot and top with the onion, garlic, lemon juice and coconut milk mixture.

Let it cook on low heat for about 6 to 8 hours until the chicken is tender.

Shred the chicken then serve alongside Garlic and basil rice (optional).

Detox Broth

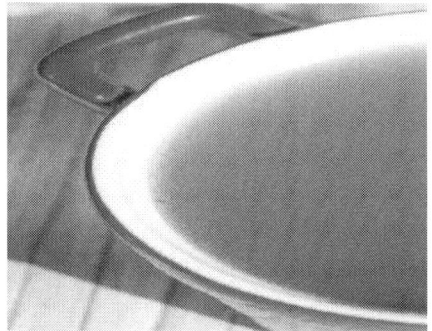

Serves 4

Ingredients

1 or 2 cups of two to five roughly chopped vegetables such as onion, cabbage, zucchini, chard with stems, kale, green beans, celery or celeriac

4 cups bone broth from an organic chicken or filtered water

Maldon sea salt to taste

½ teaspoon turmeric powder

Juice from one meyer lemon

1 tablespoon fresh herbs such as tarragon or parsley

2 tablespoons minced fresh ginger root

Directions

Place the chopped vegetables in a stock pot and pour in the bone broth or filtered water.

Add the ginger root then boil them and let them simmer for 40 minutes. Add turmeric powder, lemon juice and herbs

Strain the broth then serve.

Crunchy And Sweet Quinoa Salad

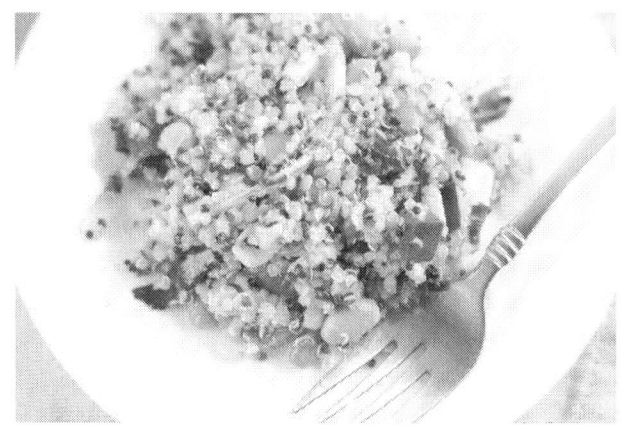

Serves 4

Ingredients

4 sliced scallions

½ teaspoon cinnamon

½ teaspoon ground cumin

¼ teaspoon ground black pepper

¼ teaspoon salt

4 teaspoons apple cider vinegar

1/3 cup pine nuts

3 separate tablespoons extra virgin oil

1 medium sweet potato, peeled and cut into ½ inch cubes

1 cup rinsed quinoa

Directions

Preheat oven to 400° F.

Pour quinoa into a small saucepan and add 2 cups of water.

Boil and let it simmer for 15 minutes or until the water evaporates. Turn off the heat and set aside to let it cool while covered for an hour.

Place sweet potato cubes in a roasting pan and toss with ½ tablespoon of olive oil. Let it bake for around 25 minutes or until you can pierce the cubes with a fork then set aside.

Place the pine nuts into a small pan over medium heat while stirring until they toast slightly then set aside.

Add the rest of the ingredients i.e. cinnamon, cumin, pepper, salt, vinegar and olive oil to a small bowl and whisk well.

After quinoa dries up, use your whisk to break the seeds apart then place them in a large bowl.

Add half of the vinaigrette and mix again with the whisk depending on how you want your quinoa to be.

Add scallions, sweet potatoes and pine nuts then mix gently.

Serve at room temperature.

White Bean Chicken Chili

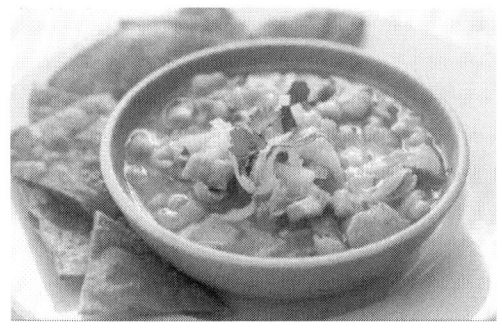

Serves 4

Ingredients

1 sliced avocado

1 cup chopped kale

1 ½ cups diced carrots

¾ cup diced celery

3 to 4 cups separate chicken broth

1 can (15 ounces) of rinsed and drained white beans

½ teaspoon ground cumin

1 teaspoon dried oregano

1 seeded and chopped jalapeno pepper

4 ounces diced mushroom

½ diced orange pepper

½ diced green pepper

2 minced garlic cloves

1 chopped medium onion

1 tablespoon olive oil

¼ teaspoon black pepper

¼ teaspoon garlic salt

2 boneless cubed skinless chicken breasts

Directions

Sprinkle the chicken with pepper and salt.

Brown the chicken in oil in a large skillet over medium heat.

Stir in the jalapeno, mushrooms, peppers, garlic and onion and cook them for two minutes.

Sprinkle in some cumin and oregano and cook for an extra minute or until the vegetables are tender and the chicken is browned. Transfer all the contents to a slow cooker.

In a small bowl, add ½ cup of chicken broth and 1 cup of beans then mash them together until they blend.

Add kale, celery, carrots, broth and beans to the slow cooker.

Cover and let it cook for 3 or 3 ½ hours, until the chicken is tender.

Stir before you serve. Garnish with sliced avocado.

Kabocha Kale Salad With Roasted Tomatillo Salmon

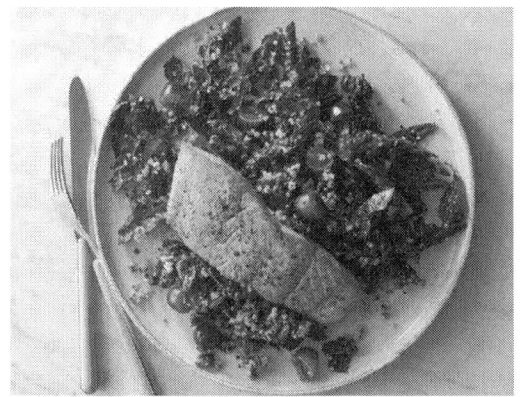

Serves 4

Ingredients for salmon

¾ teaspoon cayenne powder

1 teaspoon cumin powder

1 lemon cut into 4 thin slices

1 tablespoon olive oil

4 4 Oz. fillets of wild sockeye salmon

Ingredients for Kabocha Kale salad

2 tablespoons balsamic vinegar

¼ cup of pumpkin seeds

3 minced cloves of garlic

2 tablespoons of olive oil

1 thinly sliced Kabocha squashes

Ingredients for salsa

2 quartered cloves of garlic

½ chopped bunch of cilantro

1 small seeded and chopped jalapeno

1 peeled and chopped avocado

10 quartered and rinsed tomatillos without husks

Directions

Preheat your oven to 350° F.

In a medium saucepan, place a steamer basket with water and boil it.

Put the Kabocha in the steamer basket. Cover and let it steam for 15 to 20 minutes, until tender.

Put the salmon in a ceramic baking dish or on a baking sheet.

Brush the salmon fillets with olive oil and top every fillet with a slice of lemon. Sprinkle with a pinch of cayenne and a pinch of cumin.

Bake for about 12 minutes until it appears opaque.

As the squash steams and the salmon bakes, place the garlic, cilantro, jalapeno, avocado and tomatillos in a blender or food processor and pulse to combine. Sprinkle some sea salt to taste and set aside.

In a large skillet, heat olive oil over medium heat. Add the garlic and let it cook for 1 or 2 minutes until it begins to brown. Then add kale and sauté them while tossing time and again for 5 minutes until they wilt.

Place the salmon on a plate and top with tomatillo salsa.

Layer the kabocha squash in a pinwheel and top with kale and sprinkle with vinegar and pumpkin seeds then serve alongside the salmon.

Quinoa With Grilled Veggies

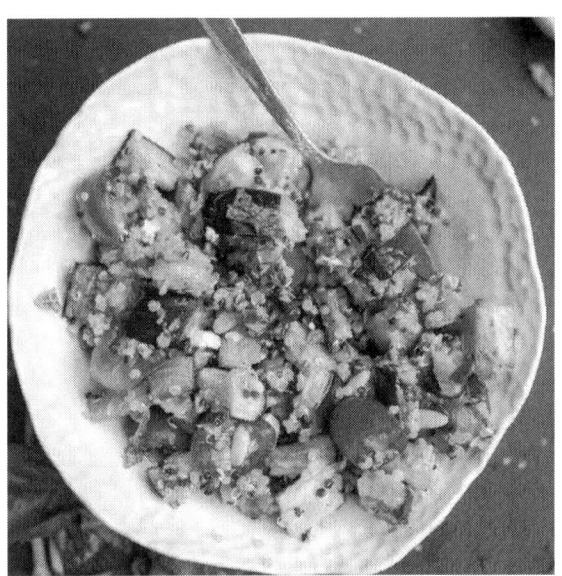

Hormone Reset Diet Meal Plan

Serves 4

Ingredients for veggies

¼ teaspoon fresh thyme

2 tablespoons extra virgin olive oil

1 large halved avocado

1 medium halved lengthwise zucchini

½ pound trimmed asparagus

1 halved large tomato

Ingredients for quinoa

½ seeded and finely diced red bell pepper

2 minced garlic cloves

2 minced shallots

1 ½ tablespoons extra virgin olive oil

2 cups quinoa, soaked for an hour and rinsed

Salt and pepper to taste

Ingredients for dressing

1 ½ tablespoons lemon juice

1 ½ tablespoons balsamic vinegar

3 ½ tablespoons extra virgin olive oil

Salt and pepper to taste

Ingredients for garnish

4 large fresh basil leaves, rolled and cut into strips

Toasted walnuts

¾ cup of kalamata olives or black olives

A bed of fresh mixed greens

Directions

Start by placing the quinoa in a large saucepan and sprinkle with slightly salted water. Cook for 15 minutes or until it is fluffy and dry. Empty to a large bowl and let it cool.

In a skillet, heat oil over medium heat then sauté the red pepper, garlic and shallots for about 5 minutes until soft. Season with pepper and salt to taste then transfer to the quinoa and mix thoroughly.

Over medium heat, heat the grill pan or grill.

Put the veggies on a baking sheet and brush them with oil. Grill them for 5 to 7 minutes. Then place them on a cutting board, add thyme and chop them into bite manageable pieces.

Put a bed of greens on a large platter and top with quinoa. Put the veggies on the quinoa and then garnish with the basil, walnuts, and olives on top.

Whisk lemon, vinegar and olive oil together and sprinkle evenly over the salad. Season with fresh black pepper and salt to taste.

Probiotic Kelp Bowl

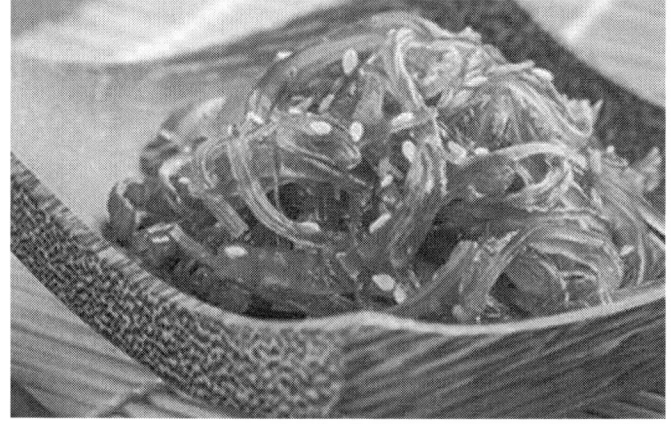

Hormone Reset Diet Meal Plan

Serves 4

Ingredients

2 to 3 teaspoons of seaweed rice seasoning blend such as Yasai Fumi Furikake

2 to 3 teaspoons of hemp or chia seeds (optional)

2 to 3 teaspoons of kelp granules

2 tablespoons (more or less) of sesame seeds (optional)

½ cup (more or less) hot chili sesame oil

¼ cup tamari

4 diced tomatillos (optional)

4 sliced hard boiled eggs

2 cups of kimchi (add more if desired)

2 sliced avocados

3 to 4 cups of cooked quinoa (or millet)

4 cups of greens of your choice

Directions

Divide the millet and greens between 4 bowls or plates.

Top each with 1 boiled egg and ¼ avocado.

Sprinkle with tomatillos and top with kimchi.

Drizzle sesame oil and tamari over each bowl.

Mix together the seaweed seasoning blend, hemp or chia seeds, kelp granules and sesame seeds and sprinkle it over the salads.

Chicken Soup And Toasted Rice With Lemon

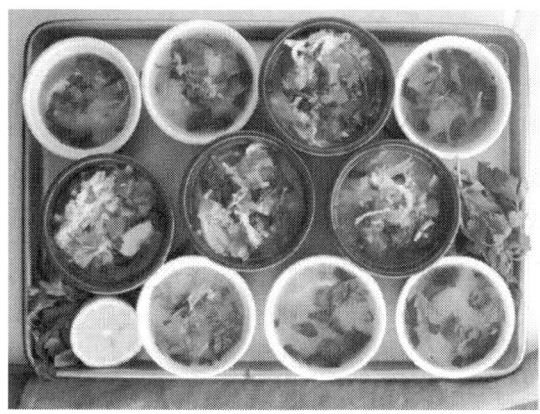

Serves 6

Ingredients

1 large skinless and boneless chicken breast

2 finely diced large celery stalks

2 finely diced large carrots

5 cups chicken broth

½ cup quick cooking brown rice

2 cups roughly chopped baby spinach

½ cup finely diced onion

Directions

Switch your instant pot to the sauté function. Add 1 tablespoon of olive oil to it.

When it heats up, add the celery, onions, carrots and rice.

Sauté for 4 or 5 minutes until the rice begins to toast slightly. If that happens, you will smell it.

Sprinkle some pepper and salt.

After the rice is toasted and the vegetables translucent, add the chicken breast. Make sure you add pepper and salt as required to both sides of the chicken breast.

Add the 5 cups of broth and cook for 7 minutes on manual high pressure after which you let a natural release to happen for 5 minutes

Remove the chicken and shred it before returning it in the pot. Stir in the baby spinach and allow them to wilt then add the lemon juice.

Garnish with parsley then serve it hot

Quinoa, Avocado And Garbanzo Bean Salad

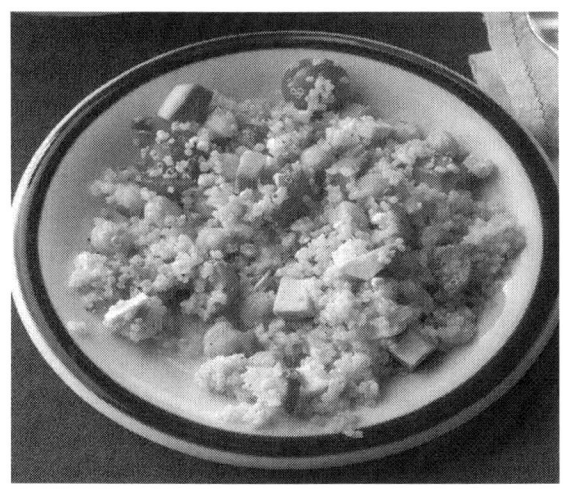

Serves 4 to 6

Ingredients

1 chopped cucumber

Pepper and salt

2 cups of cooked quinoa

Juice from 1 lemon

1 cup of halved cherry tomatoes

2 tablespoons extra virgin oil

1 large sliced avocado

1 can (15 ounces) of garbanzo beans

Directions

Toss the ingredients above in a large bowl. Mix them well and serve.

Dinner Recipes

Zucchini Lasagna And Turkey

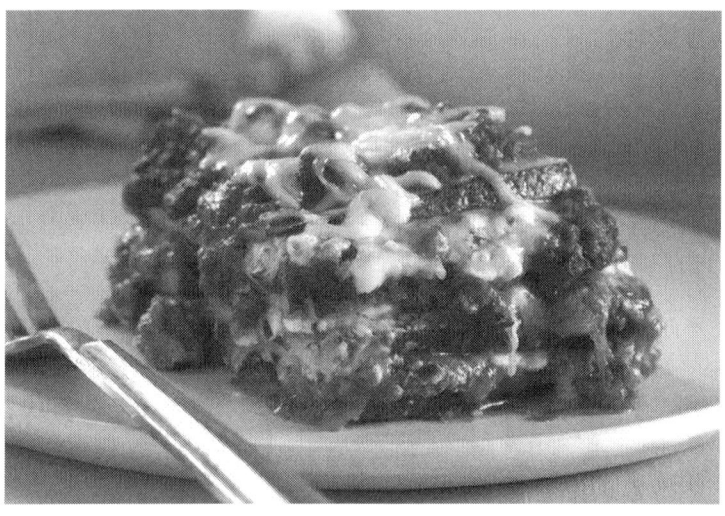

Hormone Reset Diet Meal Plan

Serves 4

Ingredients

1 can sugar free, gluten free, organic tomato sauce

1 teaspoon thyme

1 teaspoon sage

1 teaspoon rosemary

1 teaspoon dried basil

1 teaspoon oregano

4 organic egg whites

2 minced garlic cloves

1 small finely chopped yellow onion

1 teaspoon black pepper

2 separate teaspoons sea salt

6 tablespoons olive oil, divided in half

1 teaspoon garlic powder

3 tablespoons coconut milk

2 cups chopped cauliflower

1 medium finely diced green bell pepper

1 medium finely diced red bell pepper

1 8-ounce can tomato paste

5 or 6 large Zucchinis

Directions

Preheat oven to 350° F.

Use a mandolin slicer to slice Zucchinis lengthwise into very thin strips. Sprinkle each with salt and set aside.

In a large skillet, heat 3 tablespoons of olive oil over medium heat. Add garlic and onion then sauté until translucent

Stir in the ground turkey and cook for about 4 minutes.

Add all bell peppers and herbs and keep cooking until the peppers are soft and turkey is brown then add tomato sauce and mix well. Remove from heat and set aside.

Boil or steam the cauliflower until tender. Place the cauliflower in a blender with coconut milk, garlic powder, pepper, salt and 3 tablespoons of olive oil. Blend until creamy and smooth and add more coconut milk if necessary.

Spray coconut oil or non-stick olive oil onto a deep 8 by 8 inch baking dish.

Line the zucchinis on the bottom of the baking dish. Ensure each zucchini strip overlaps slightly. Add a thin layer of turkey mixture on the zucchinis. Cover the layer with tomato sauce then add a ¼ inch thick layer of the cauliflower.

Repeat the layering of zucchini, turkey, tomato sauce and cauliflower as many times as you wish then finish off with a layer of tomato sauce.

Whisk egg whites until frothy and pour on the lasagna evenly.

Bake for 20 or 30 minutes at 350° F or until the eggs are set.

Serve and enjoy.

Cauliflower Soup

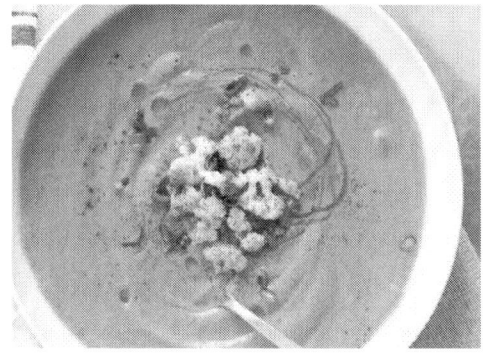

Serves 4 to 6

Ingredients

1 head cauliflower cut into florets

2 tablespoons tahini

4 cups organic chicken stock

1 russet potato cut into 1 inch cubes

1 clove minced garlic

1 medium coarsely chopped onion

1 tablespoon olive oil

Slivered almonds to garnish

Salt and pepper to taste

Directions

In a large pot, heat oil over medium heat then sauté the garlic and onions for 5 minutes, until the onions appear translucent.

Add the potato and cauliflower and keep cooking for 3 more minutes.

Add chicken stock then boil them and afterwards reduce the heat and simmer for 20 to 25 minutes until the potato is tender.

Add tahini then using an immersion blender, blend the soup until velvety and smooth. Alternatively, you can transfer to a blender and puree.

Season with pepper and salt then garnish with almonds. For a more vibrant flavor, toast the almonds first.

Stuffed Mushrooms

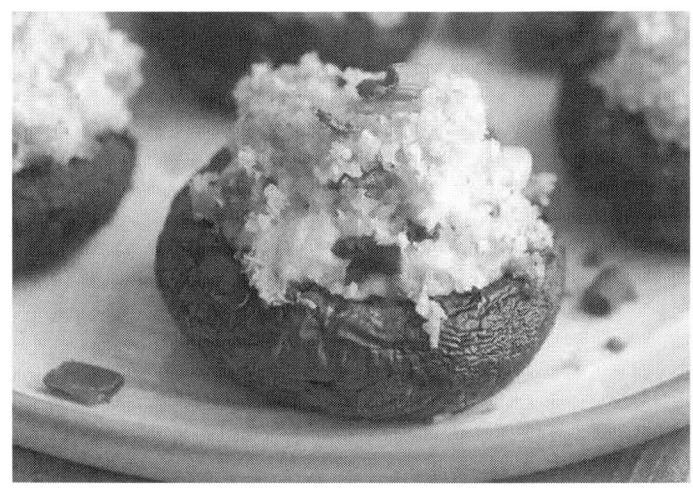

Serves 4

Ingredients

4 Portobello mushrooms

1 ripe avocado

2 tablespoons fresh lemon juice

5 tablespoons nutritional yeast

¼ cup pecans

2 cloves garlic

1 cup packed baby spinach

2 separate tablespoons coconut oil

Pinch of cayenne pepper

Black pepper and sea salt to taste

Directions

Preheat oven to 450° F.

Wipe the mushrooms with a damp towel paper to remove the stem. Brush the top of the mushroom with a tablespoon of coconut oil and place the cap side down on a baking sheet. Sprinkle some sea salt.

Let it bake for 8 minutes then pour the liquid out of the caps and put back onto the baking sheet.

Put the rest of the ingredients (except the avocado) in a food processor and puree until smooth to make the filling.

Peel and pit the avocado then mash it with a fork to leave some chunks.

Mix the chunky avocado and the filling and add a pinch of cayenne pepper, black pepper and sea salt then taste.

Spoon the filling into the mushrooms and warm in the oven for 5 minutes then serve.

Tahini Roasted Whole Cauliflower

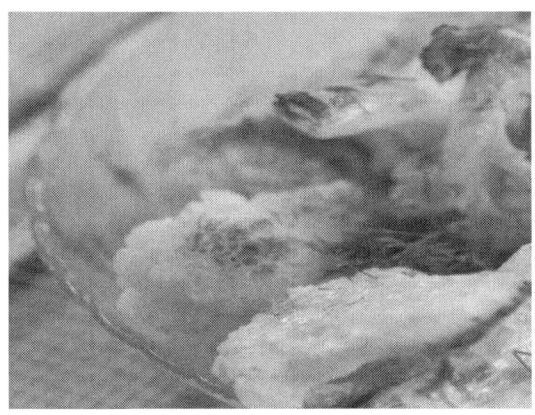

Serves 4

Ingredients

1 head of cauliflower without the leaves

½ teaspoon garlic powder

¼ teaspoon cumin

Juice and zest of 1 lemon

1 cup tahini

Pepper and salt to taste

Directions

Preheat oven to 400° F.

Wash the cauliflower, cut at bottom level and remove the leaves.

Mix tahini with pepper and salt, garlic powder, cumin, lemon zest and juice in a small bowl.

Line a baking sheet with foil or parchment paper. Drizzle grape seed oil or olive oil on the pan to avoid the cauliflower from sticking.

Massage the tahini mixture over the cauliflower. If any marinade is left over, you can use it as a dip or a salad dressing later on.

Roast the cauliflower for about 40 minutes or until it tender.

Spicy Tuna Bowl With Vegetables

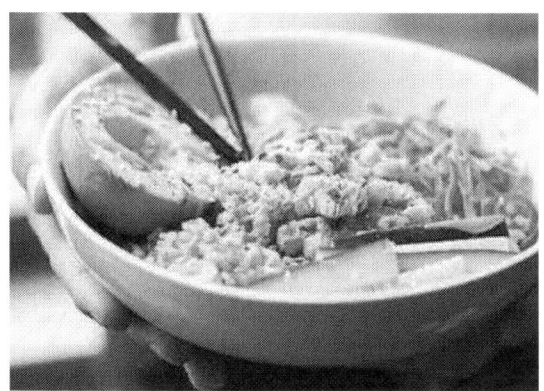

Serves 4

Ingredients

2 julienned or sliced Jerusalem artichokes and/or carrots

2 quartered avocadoes

3 tablespoons sesame seeds

16 - 20 ounces sushi grade Ahi tuna

Cilantro to taste

¼ cup chopped cilantro

1 tablespoon lime or lemon juice

1 cup of diced red bell pepper

2 cups chopped cabbage (preferably a mixture of Napa and purple varieties)

Directions

Make a curtado by tossing the ingredients together in a bowl.

Coat the edge of the tuna in sesame seeds.

Slide the tuna into small quarters about 1 by 2 inches in size.

Spray a hot pan with coconut oil and cook the tuna lightly in the hot pan.

Assemble each bowl. At the bottom begin with the vegetables Jerusalem artichokes or carrots, then add avocado to one side, tuna to the other side and top off with the curtado

Cilantro Pesto And Zucchini Noodles

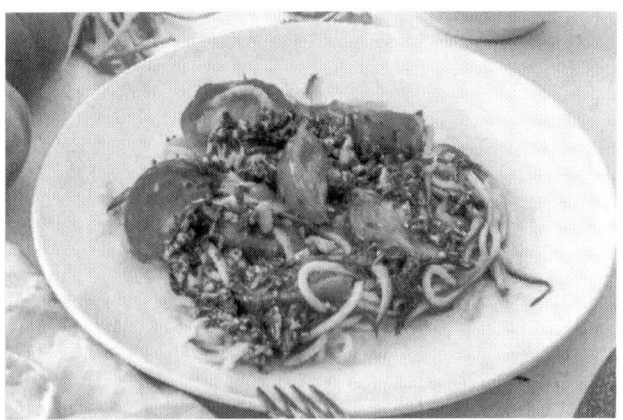

Serves 2

Ingredients for zucchini noodles

2 sliced heirloom tomatoes

1 tablespoon olive oil

2 large zucchini

Pinch of salt

Ingredients for cilantro pesto

¼ cup olive oil

1 bunch cilantro

¼ teaspoon salt

¼ cup pine nuts

2 to 3 cloves minced garlic

Juice from ½ lemon

Directions

Add the pine nuts, garlic, lemon juice, olive oil, cilantro and salt in a food processor and pulse until finely chopped. You could also use a mortar and pestle to grind further and release the flavors.

Chop the ends of the zucchini such that both sides are flat. Fasten them to a spiralizer using the thin julienne blade to make noodles.

In a skillet, heat olive oil over medium heat. Add the sliced heirloom tomatoes and zucchini noodles. Heat and toss for about 3 to 5 minutes until they noodles are tender but still holding shape. Sprinkle some salt.

Top the heirloom tomatoes and zucchini noodles with the cilantro pesto and serve immediately.

Spiralized Sweet Potato Salad With Pesto

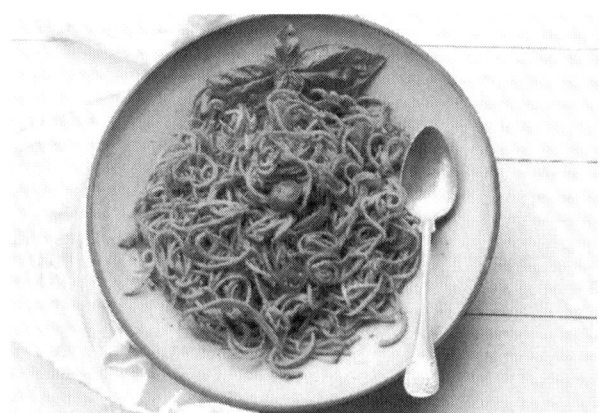

Serves 8

Ingredients

2 small, peeled sweet potatoes

1 or 2 tablespoons water

¼ cup vegan pesto regular subs

¼ cup halved cherry tomatoes

1 tablespoon coconut oil

1 large zucchini

Directions

Spiralize the zucchini and sweet potatoes on small spaghetti setting. In a sauté pan, cook the sweet potatoes in coconut oil over medium heat for about 10 minutes until tender.

Add the zucchini and cook again for about 3 or 4 minutes until soft then transfer to a mixing bowl.

Combine pesto with water to thin the pesto for use as a dressing. Pour it into the mixing bowl with the cherry tomatoes.

Toss the sweet potato mixture in dressing and serve.

Cauliflower Fried Rice

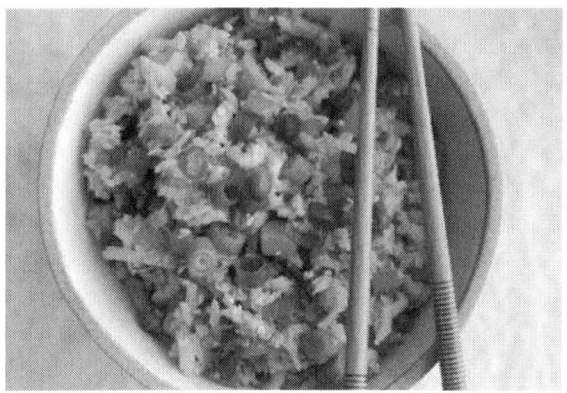

Serves 4

Ingredients

4 sliced scallions with green and white parts separated

2 garlic cloves

2 large eggs

2 tablespoons coconut aminos or tamari

1 large or 2 to 3 small carrots sliced into small bits

2 tablespoons sesame oil

1 medium head of cauliflower

½ teaspoon of minced ginger

½ cup of frozen peas, thawed

½ small diced onion

Directions

Slice the head of the cauliflower into two equal halves, then slice off the florets from the stem. Place the florets through the grater of a food processor and process until all cauliflower has been 'riced'.

Heat sesame oil on medium heat in a skillet or huge wok.

Add ginger and garlic then sauté for 20 seconds.

Stir in the carrots, onions and white parts of the scallions and let it cook for 3 minutes.

Add peas and cauliflower rice and stir for another 2 or 3 minutes.

Create a well in the middle of the rice and break the eggs inside the well.

Stir with a spatula to scramble the eggs.

Once the eggs are cooked, stir everything together.

Finally add the green parts of the scallion and tamari then stir to combine.

Serve while hot.

Avocado Couscous Salad

Serves 6

Ingredients

100g toasted pine nuts

1 tablespoon flat of chopped leaf parsley

2 tablespoons chopped mint

2 tablespoons virgin olive oil

4 tablespoons orange juice

1 pomegranate

1 finely chopped red pepper

1 220g drained can of chickpeas

1 tablespoon lemon juice

500g couscous 2 avocados

Directions

Cover the couscous with boiled water and cover with a damp tea cloth. Leave it there to soak for 20 minutes then fork through to loosen the grains.

Peel and stone the avocado. Cut it into chunks and squeeze in the lemon juice.

Mix together the pepper, chickpeas and avocado and add it to the couscous.

Split the pomegranate over a bowl to catch any juices and remove its seeds.

Add the seeds to the couscous.

Mix the olive oil, lemon juice and orange juice and whisk them.

Add the herbs and dressing to the couscous and fork through.

Serve with a sprinkling of pine nuts.

Oven Baked Sweet Potato Fries

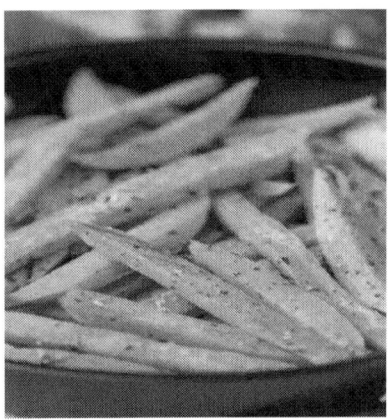

Serves 6

Ingredients

1 tablespoon organic coconut oil

2 large sweet potatoes

Pinch of cayenne pepper

¼ teaspoon trace mineral salt or sea salt

Directions

Preheat your oven to 425° F.

Toss the potato wedges with sea salt, coconut oil and cayenne pepper.

Spread out the sweet potato wedges out on a rimmed baking sheet.

Put them in the oven and bake them for about 20 minutes until they are tender and brown.

Serve when hot.

Chicken Curry In A Hurry

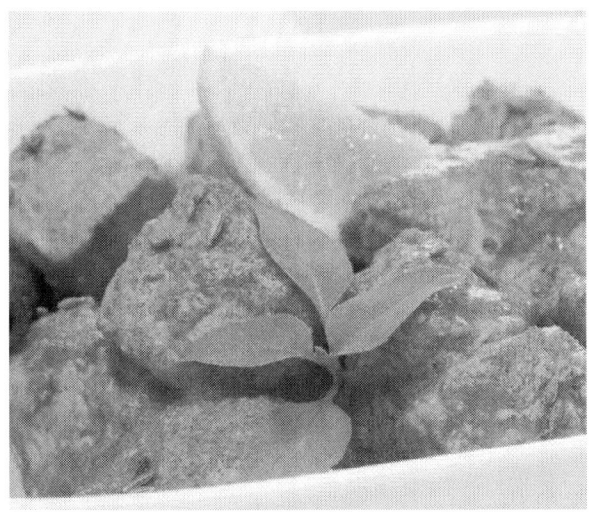

Serves 2 or 3

Ingredients

2 handfuls spinach

½ head cabbage

4 heads bok choy

1 onion

3 tablespoons curry paste

1 cup chicken broth (or filtered water) with some sea salt

1 BPA free can of coconut milk

1 pound of boneless chicken thighs

Directions

Pour the broth and coconut milk in a crock pot.

Add the curry paste then stir until coconut milk dissolves.

Cut the chicken thighs into 1 inch pieces and put them in the pot.

Chop all the vegetables into bit sized pieces and put them in the pot as well.

Cover the pot and cook on low heat for 4 hours.

Set aside and garnish with a tablespoon of grated ginger, a squeeze of fresh lemon and fresh cilantro for a more kick.

Now that we have lots of mouthwatering recipes that you can prepare to reset your hormones, let's put it all together in a way that you can actually follow to see your hormones reset in as little as 21 days!

21 Day Hormone Reset Plan

WEEK 1		
MONDAY	BREAKFAST	Vanilla green milkshake
	LUNCH	Garlic and basil rice
	DINNER	Zucchini lasagna and Turkey
TUESDAY	BREAKFAST	Kraut and eggs
	LUNCH	Roasted beets and greens gluten free pasta
	DINNER	Cauliflower soup
WEDNESDAY	BREAKFAST	Nutty seed granola
	LUNCH	Lemon chicken with Crockpot coconut
	DINNER	Stuffed mushrooms
THURSDAY	BREAKFAST	Berry and coconut smoothie

Hormone Reset Diet Meal Plan

	LUNCH	Detox broth
	DINNER	Tahini Roasted Whole Cauliflower
FRIDAY	BREAKFAST	Farmer's wife breakfast
	LUNCH	Crunchy and sweet quinoa salad
	DINNER	Spicy tuna bowl with vegetables
SATURDAY	BREAKFAST	Ginger rhubarb cider
	LUNCH	White bean chicken chili
	DINNER	Cilantro pesto and zucchini noodles
SUNDAY	BREAKFAST	Posh beans on toast
	LUNCH	Kabocha Kale salad with roasted Tomatillo Salmon
	DINNER	Spiralized sweet potato salad with pesto

Hormone Reset Diet Meal Plan

	WEEK 2	
MONDAY	BREAKFAST	Raw chocolate chia pancakes
	LUNCH	Quinoa with grilled veggies
	DINNER	Avocado couscous salad
TUESDAY	BREAKFAST	Collagen frappe and tea
	LUNCH	Probiotic kelp bowl
	DINNER	Savory shake
WEDNESDAY	BREAKFAST	Healthy egg, ham and chips
	LUNCH	Chicken soup and toasted rice with lemon
	DINNER	Oven baked sweet potato fries
THURSDAY	BREAKFAST	Chocolate dipped

Hormone Reset Diet Meal Plan

			banana bites
	LUNCH		Quinoa, avocado and garbanzo bean salad
	DINNER		Chicken curry in a hurry
FRIDAY	BREAKFAST		Sweet spirit
	LUNCH		Chicken soup and toasted rice with lemon
	DINNER		Cauliflower fried rice
SATURDAY	BREAKFAST		Farmer's wife breakfast
	LUNCH		Probiotic kelp bowl
	DINNER		Spicy tuna bowl with vegetables
SUNDAY	BREAKFAST		Kraut and eggs
	LUNCH		Quinoa with grilled veggies
	DINNER		Avocado couscous salad

WEEK 3

MONDAY	BREAKFAST	Kale and sunflower smoothie
	LUNCH	White bean chicken chili
	DINNER	Spiralized sweet potato salad with pesto
TUESDAY	BREAKFAST	Raw chocolate chia pancakes
	LUNCH	Kabocha Kale salad with roasted Tomatillo Salmon
	DINNER	Stuffed mushrooms
WEDNESDAY	BREAKFAST	Healthy egg, ham and chips
	LUNCH	Crunchy and sweet quinoa salad
	DINNER	Oven baked sweet potato fries

Hormone Reset Diet Meal Plan

THURSDAY	BREAKFAST	Adaptogenic tea
	LUNCH	Detox broth
	DINNER	Cilantro pesto and zucchini noodles
FRIDAY	BREAKFAST	Posh beans on toast
	LUNCH	Lemon chicken with Crockpot coconut
	DINNER	Tahini Roasted Whole Cauliflower
SATURDAY	BREAKFAST	Nutty seed granola
	LUNCH	Roasted beets and greens gluten free pasta
	DINNER	Chicken curry in a hurry
SUNDAY	BREAKFAST	Ginger rhubarb cider
	LUNCH	Garlic and basil rice
	DINNER	Zucchini lasagna and Turkey

Conclusion

The Hormone Reset Diet is a professionally designed detoxification plan and is an effective hit-the-reset-button for your hormones. It will enable you to feel and look your best each and every day. By following it, you can finally shed unwanted body fat, restore your hormones and health, rediscover the body you always dream about and feel fit and sexy. You can do it.

Printed in Great Britain
by Amazon